Microsurgical Reconstruction
of the Extremities

Microsurgical Reconstruction of the Extremities

Indications, Technique, and Postoperative Care

Leonard Gordon, M.B.B.Ch.

Associate Clinical Professor of Orthopaedic Surgery
Lecturer, Department of Anatomy
University of California, San Francisco

Illustrations by James Brodale and Susan Taft

With 135 Figures in 538 Parts, 156 in Color

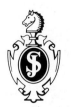

Springer-Verlag
New York Berlin Heidelberg
London Paris Tokyo

LEONARD GORDON, M.B.B.CH.
Director, Hand and Microsurgery Service, Department of Orthopaedic Surgery,
University of California, San Francisco and Mt. Zion Hospital Medical Center
Microsurgery Consultant, Oak Knoll Naval Base and Letterman Army Medical
Center

Library of Congress Cataloging-in-Publication Data
Gordon, Leonard
Microsurgical reconstruction of the extremities.
Includes bibliographies and index.
1. Extremities (Anatomy) – Surgery. 2. Microsurgery.
3. Extremities (Anatomy) – Transplantation.
4. Postoperative care. I. Title. [DNLM: 1. Extremities
– transplantation. 2. Microsurgery – methods.
3. Postoperative Care. 4. Replantation. WE 800 G663 m]
RD551.G65   1988   617'.58059   87-32362

Typeset, printed, and bound by Universitätsdruckerei H. Stürtz AG, Würzburg, Federal
Republic of Germany.

9 8 7 6 5 4 3 2 1

ISBN 0-387-96632-3 Springer-Verlag New York Berlin Heidelberg
ISBN 3-540-96632-3 Springer-Verlag Berlin Heidelberg New York

*To my wife Chandra
and "the boys" –
Danny, Josh, and Coby,*

and

*in memory of
my friend and teacher,
Richard J. Smith, M.D.*

Preface

The purpose of this book is to provide the extremity surgeon with practical information on microvascular repair and reconstruction. To be successful, the surgeon performing a microvascular procedure must have an intimate knowledge of vascular anatomy and be able to apply this knowledge in performing a meticulous surgical dissection. Unfortunately, the anatomy required for microvascular procedures is not found in standard anatomy texts or atlases because many of the vessels used in microvascular procedures have not previously been regarded as having great anatomic importance. This book evolved from the repeated requests of residents and fellows for clarification on points of anatomy and surgical dissection as they prepared for microvascular procedures.

A thorough knowledge of the various procedures that can be used to treat a particular clinical problem is equally important. Options must necessarily include well-established nonmicrosurgical techniques as well as an analysis and comparison of the various microsurgical alternatives. Each surgeon must establish his or her own philosophy for the use of these procedures. One such approach is given here.

A microsurgical armamentarium is presented which will allow the care of almost any clinical problem where microsurgical technique may be appropriate. With this in mind, transplants of various tissues and sizes are described. There are many microvascular procedures that have not been included, and I have done my best to provide a rationale behind procedure selection. Each surgeon will necessarily prefer certain procedures over others, and no surgeon will use all of the transplants available. This practice is to be encouraged to foster proficiency. Reconstructive possibilities are limited only by the imagination and skills of the surgeon, and my hope is that this text will be used as a foundation on which each practitioner can build.

The bibliographies consist of only those journal articles that deal with indications and surgical technique. Many outstanding contributions have not been included to avoid duplication of information and to make the text as simple to use as possible. Toward this end, each entry includes a brief description to help the reader determine whether a detailed study of the article will be valuable.

Tissue survival rates of over 95% should be attained. This can only be accomplished by first mastering the techniques of microsurgical anastomosis in the laboratory. There are many practical courses and texts that offer detailed instruction, but there is no substitute for the many hours of laboratory practice required to perfect these techniques. Combining meticulous microsurgical technique with appropriate cadaver dissections to prepare for these procedures, and having a clear understanding of the indications and postoperative program will ensure a successful outcome.

LEONARD GORDON

Acknowledgements

In our specialized world, most endeavors require a team approach. Both the successful outcomes of the microsurgical procedures documented herein and the presentation of this text are evidence of this. Neither would have been possible without the immense contributions of many in the Department of Orthopaedic Surgery at the University of California, San Francisco.

The bibliography of microsurgery was electronically compiled by Elaine Chiu, who made possible the review and selection of articles. I thank her for obtaining and helping to summarize each of these papers, as well as for assisting in the anatomic cadaver dissections. The enormous editing project was ably done by Judith Simon. Microsurgeons performing these procedures would do well to adopt her meticulous attention to detail. Jackie Benson deserves my special thanks and appreciation for her prodigious effort in typing, retyping, and printing out the many drafts of the manuscript. I also wish to compliment Chong Lee and Ellen Caruthers for producing the hundreds of excellent black-and-white prints.

All of the patients presented in this book are from my personal practice except the two provided by Hill Hastings II, M.D. I greatly appreciate his contributing these outstanding cases which illustrate the wrap-around procedure and the radial forearm flap. I am indebted to Enrique Monsanto, M.D. who was an able cosurgeon for most of the cases presented in the surgical technique sections, and I extend praise and thanks to Pam Silverman, O.T.R./A.S.H.T., both for her contribution to the text and the excellent therapy she has provided to almost all of the patients presented. The University of California, San Francisco operating room team and recovery room and ward nurses are also to be commended for their fastidious care of these patients.

I am grateful to Dr. William Murray and the orthopaedic faculty for their support of the Hand and Microsurgery Service, and to the many residents who helped in these procedures. Finally, I thank my many teachers and colleagues who have shared their knowledge and inventiveness. In so doing, they have established our current fund of knowledge and ensured the continued prolific growth of microsurgery.

Contents

1
Muscle Transplantation

1.1 Overview

Muscle tissue is composed of closely packed bundles of fibers which are separated by connective tissue. Blood vessels run through these connective tissue septa and branch out to form a generous capillary network among the individual muscle fibers. This superior vascularity of muscle tissue combined with its density and ability to contour and fill "dead space" appear to make it better than skin with subcutaneous fat for treating the various clinical problems described in this chapter.

Initially, muscle pedicle flaps were the only method of transferring muscle tissue, but with this technique, a muscle cannot be moved beyond its arc of rotation without compromising its vascular and nerve supply. The advent of microsurgical muscle transplantation has expanded the versatility of muscle tissue transfer, and muscles of various sizes can now be placed in almost any anatomic location.

Four muscle transplants are described in this chapter – the *latissimus dorsi*, the *gracilis*, the lowest digitations of the *serratus anterior*, and the *tensor fasciae latae*. These four muscles can effectively treat almost any wound requiring muscle tissue because they can provide the full range of sizes and shapes that may be required.

The *latissimus dorsi* and underlying *serratus anterior* have a common proximal vascular pedicle, which makes the approach to harvesting these two muscles similar. Either the latissimus dorsi, the lowest digitations of the serratus anterior, or both can be harvested (Harii et al. 1982). They may also be used where there is a large dead space. This dead space can be filled by the serratus anterior with the overlying latissimus used for soft-tissue cover. The serratus anterior is small and flat, whereas the latissimus dorsi is large and flat and can cover extremely extensive soft-tissue wounds. The *gracilis* is intermediate in size, longer, and somewhat cylindrical for long and narrow wounds. The *tensor fasciae latae* is a large bulky muscle used as a muscu-

locutaneous transplant (Fig. 1-1). It can fill large defects, but its principal advantage lies in the cutaneous sensation it can provide with the lateral femoral cutaneous nerve.

1.2 Indications

1.2.1 Wound Coverage (May et al. 1984, Swartz and Mears 1985)

Muscle tissue is effective in covering wounds complicated by infection. The mechanism involved remains unclear, but as mentioned above, it may relate to the excellent vascularity of muscle, its density, and its ability to contour and fill the wound's dead space. These characteristics make it ideal for covering wounds of the following kind.

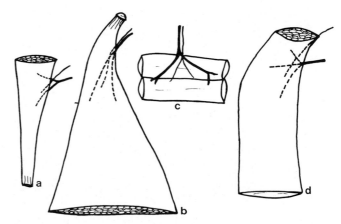

Fig. 1-1 a–d. The relative sizes and shapes of various muscle transplants are shown. **a.** Gracilis: 5 × 20 cm. **b.** Latissimus dorsi: 15 × 25–30 cm. **c.** Serratus anterior: 2 × 8 cm (each digitation). **d.** Tensor fasciae latae: 8 × 25 cm.

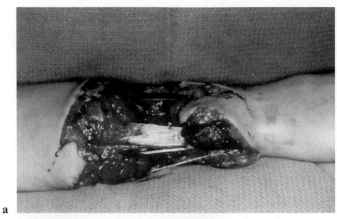

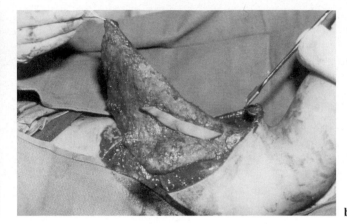

a   b

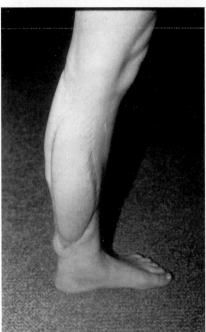

Fig. 1-2. a. An 11-year-old girl sustained an accidental gunshot wound in the left calf. The Achilles tendon was exposed, as was the posterior tibial neurovascular bundle in the depths of the wound. **b.** A latissimus dorsi muscle transplant was dissected; a small island of skin was left on the superficial surface for monitoring and was later removed. (This provision is optional because muscle tissue can be easily monitored by direct observation [Chapter 8].) **c.** The contour of the calf has been restored, although it is bulky. Excess mass can be reduced by subsequent debulking.

c

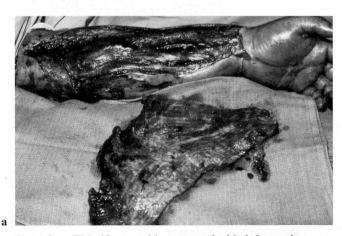

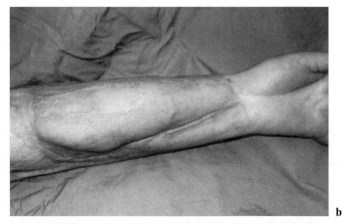

a   b

Fig. 1-3. a. This 32-year-old man caught his left arm between two rollers of a press and was trapped in this position for 8 hours. He was referred at 6 weeks with unstable fractures, delayed soft-tissue healing, and infection. The wound was debrided and the forearm bones were plated. Because of continued infection and the size of the wound, a latissimus dorsi muscle transplant was chosen. The latissimus muscle can be seen ready to cover the wound. **b.** Six months later, excellent cover had been achieved with a split-thickness skin graft used over the latissimus dorsi, and good pinch had been restored in his hand.

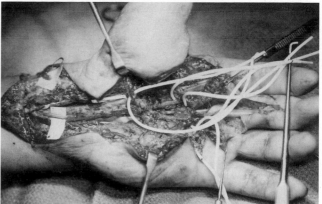

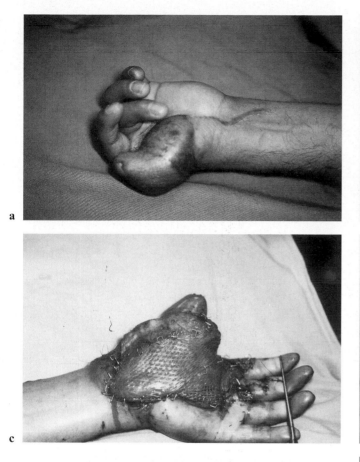

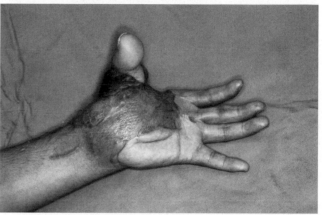

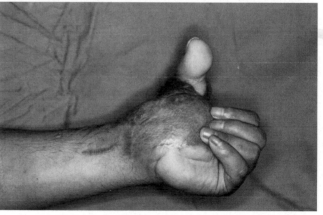

Fig. 1-4. a. This laborer sustained a saw injury across his palm along with amputation of his thumb. A pedicle groin flap had been applied around the thumb. This photograph shows his poor finger extension due to severe scarring in the palm. He also had a fixed adduction contracture of the thumb amputation stump. The hand was functionless. **b.** After releasing the contracture and all of the soft tissues of the palm, fingers, and thumb, an extensive defect remained. **c.** The serratus anterior muscle was placed in the palm and covered with a split-thickness skin graft. **d** and **e.** Six months later, a toe transplant was performed. The patient maintained excellent extension of all his fingers as well as good flexion of all but the long finger, which he learned to trap with the ring finger (he usually wore a buddy tape between the long and ring fingers). The serratus anterior provided a good palmar surface.

1.2.1.1 Traumatic Wounds – Acute Stage (Within the First Week of Injury) (Byrd et al. 1985, Godina 1986, Swartz and Mears 1985).

Extensive acute wounds in the *lower extremity* (Sec. 6.1.4-6), if covered with transplanted muscle after thorough debridement, will usually heal within a few weeks. The infection rate is extremely low, and the advantage the procedure offers through prompt healing and enabling early bone grafting is substantial (Figs. 1-2 and 3-4). In the *upper extremity* (Sec. 6.1.1-3), *smaller wounds* in which local flaps are inadequate are often amenable to standard groin or abdominal pedicle flaps.

However, after severe trauma or in other situations where hand stiffness and edema are major problems, microvascular transplantation is needed to allow early elevation of the extremity and mobilization of the joints. Cutaneous microvascular flaps such as the lateral arm and scapular flaps are indicated in such situations (Sec. 2.1, 2.3). More *extensive wounds* or those with marked potential for infection should be treated by muscle transplantation (Fig. 1-3). A serratus anterior muscle transplant covered with skin grafts is effective in covering the *palm* (Sec. 6.1.1, 1.5.2.1) because it results in less shearing of the transplant on the deeper tissues compared with cutaneous flaps (Fig. 1-4). These

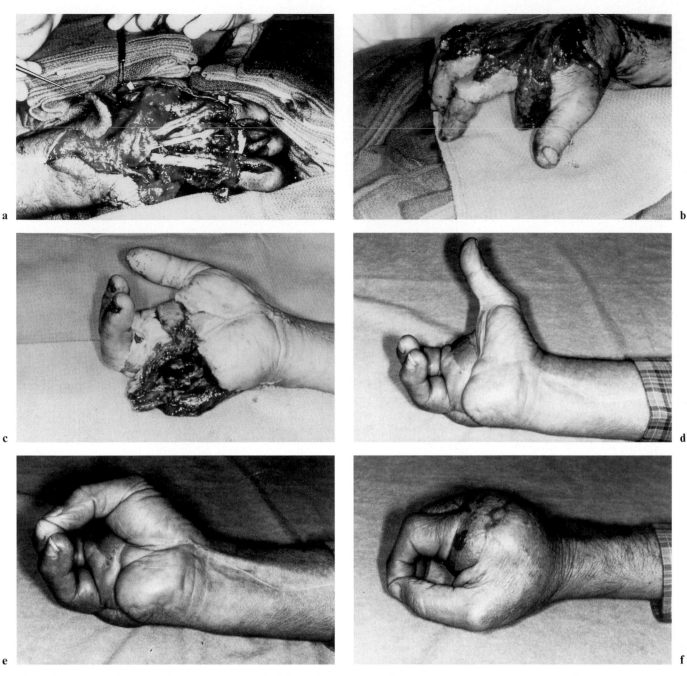

Fig. 1-5. a. This laborer suffered a severe crush injury that resulted in a hand wound requiring extensive soft-tissue reconstruction of both the palmar and dorsal surfaces. **b.** Two slips of the serratus anterior were separated to provide the dorsal cover; the third slip (the largest slip) was routed across the first web space to provide cover in the palm. **c.** The patient ultimately lost his ring and small fingers because of vascular problems, but the muscle provided excellent soft-tissue cover on both sides of the hand. **d–f.** Ultimate function was good for both large and small object grasp.

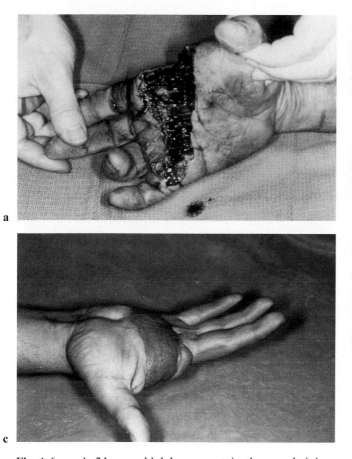

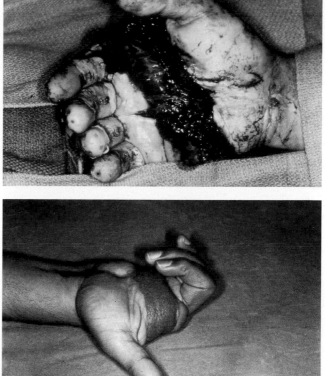

a
b
c
d

Fig. 1-6. a. A 24-year-old laborer sustained a crush injury to his palm with devascularization of the index, long, and ring fingers. Vein grafting was required. **b.** There was substantial necrosis of palmar skin, exposing the vein grafts, tendons, and nerves. One week after the injury, a single slip of the serratus anterior was used across the palm to provide good vascularized cover; this in turn was covered with a split-thick- ness skin graft. A ray amputation of the index finger had to be performed because vascularity could not be maintained. **c** and **d.** Subsequently, tendon and nerve grafting were required; this restored good flexion of the fingers. The palmar skin has proved to be a durable surface, and the patient continues to work as a laborer 3 years later.

muscle slips are particularly useful if the cover must be "tailored" to the contour of the defect. This need occurs in multiple digit wounds (Figs. 1-5 and 1-6) or those involving both the palm and dorsum of the hand (Fig. 1-7). Tendon reconstruction beneath a serratus transplant to the hand generally requires silicone tendon rods. Placement of these rods, which can sometimes be performed at the time of the muscle transplant, is done as the first of a two-stage reconstruction. On the *dorsum of the hand* (Sec. 6.1.1), cutaneous transplants are preferable because they more closely simulate the pliable skin of this region, especially if subsequent tendon reconstruction is anticipated. For extensive defects of the palm and dorsum, where attempts at hand salvage are appropriate, a combination latissimus dorsi and serratus anterior transplant can be used (Fig. 1-8).

The *timing* of debridement and flap coverage is of the utmost importance. If treated within a week of injury, wounds have the lowest rate of infection and flaps have the highest rate of success. Meticulously thorough debridement of the entire wound is essential. The margins and base of the wound should be sharply debrided back to healthy tissue. After this stage, the tissues, including the recipient vessels, become increasingly edematous and inflamed. There are two situations in which performing a flap in the acute stage is unwise: when a patient's general condition makes major surgery risky, and when the extent of tissue necrosis cannot be assessed.

If a flap cannot be done early, some surgeons advocate placing temporary skin grafts to allow as much healing as possible until the inflammation and swelling have subsided. This generally takes 6–8 weeks, at which time the microvascular flap can be safely done. Of course, the decision to perform such a flap involves many clinical factors, and if bone, nerve, or tendons are exposed, a transplant may be necessary even in the presence of swelling. If so, particular care must be taken to use recipient vessels well outside the zone of injury. (Godina et al. [1986] described "banking" an amputated hand for several months by connecting the vessels of the hand to the thoracodorsal vessels in the axilla while burns in the more proximal part of the extremity could be evaluated and treated.)

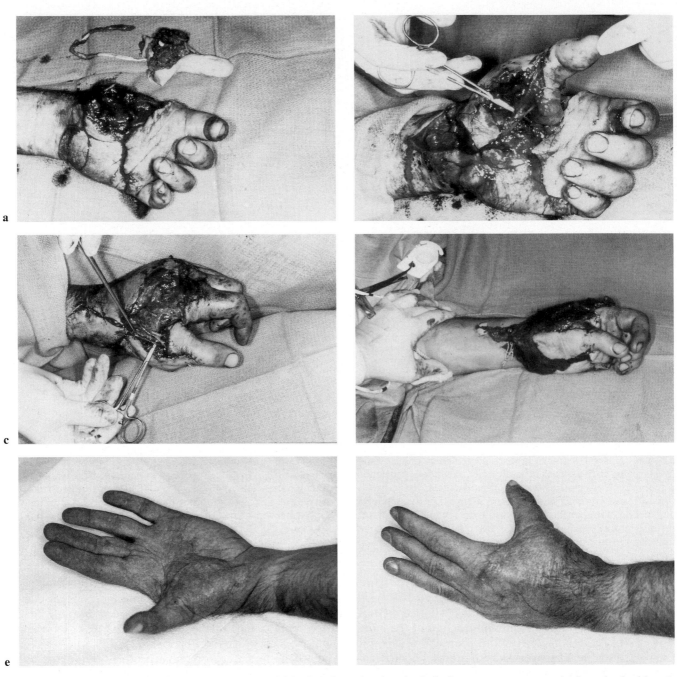

Fig. 1-7. a. This patient sustained an avulsion of his thumb and thenar eminence in a motor racing accident. **b.** The thumb was revascularized with vein grafts to replace the damaged artery, and the flexor tendon and nerves were repaired. **c.** Vein grafts were also used to reconstruct venous outflow, and the extensor tendons were repaired on the dorsum of the thumb. Soft-tissue cover was required on both sides. **d.** The serratus anterior pedicle was hooked into the radial artery with slips brought around the thumb on the palmar and dorsal surfaces. **e** and **f.** Excellent cover was achieved along with good function. The muscle, which was covered with split-thickness skin graft, has flattened out.

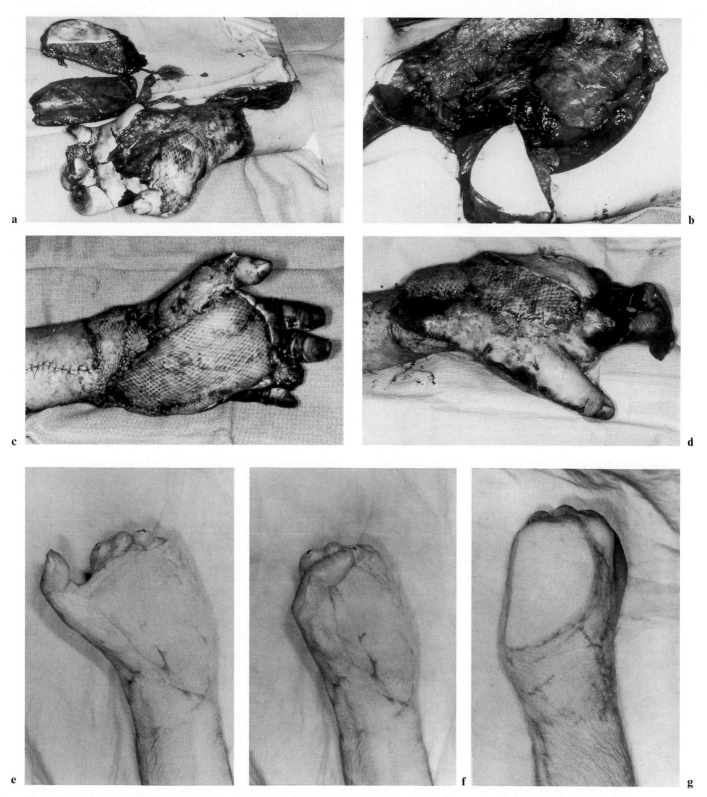

Fig. 1-8. a. A 31-year-old man crushed his hand in an industrial machine, devascularizing all of the fingers and the palm. The thumb was revascularized. Cover of the dorsum and palm was needed to salvage the hand. A combined latissimus dorsi-serratus anterior muscle transplant based on the thoracodorsal vessels was dissected from the right thorax. **b.** The combined transplant can be seen prior to its removal from the chest. **c** and **d.** The transplant was anastomosed into the ulnar vessels end-to-side, using the serratus anterior for cover on the palm and the latissimus dorsi musculocutaneous portion for the dorsum. All of the fingers became necrotic and were amputated. **e–g.** The patient regained thumb function and good cover on both the dorsum and palm. Subsequent toe transplantation was done to provide an opposable digit (Fig. 4–14).

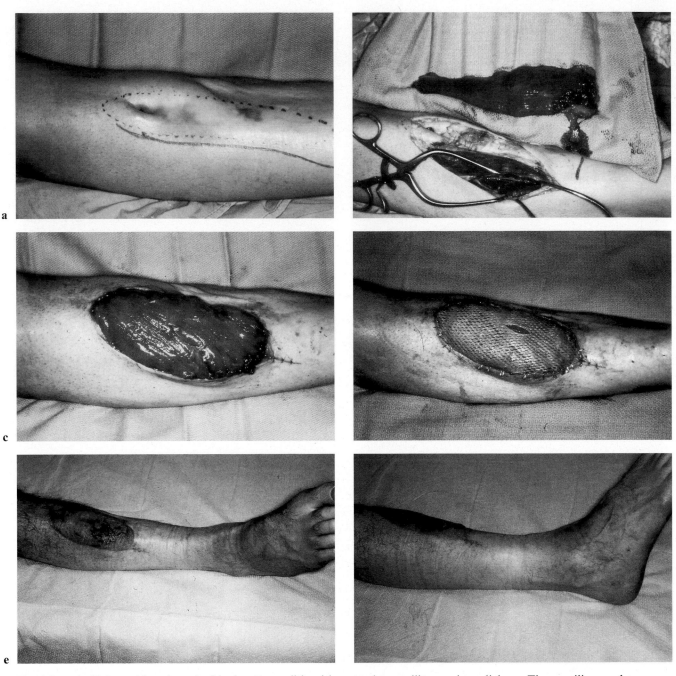

Fig. 1-9. a. A 46-year-old engineer had had osteomyelitis with repeated drainage and intermittent swelling subsequent to a tibial fracture sustained 17 years earlier. The anterior part of the leg was unsightly and the skin continually broke down. **b.** The scarred soft tissues were removed and the bone was curetted to prepare the defect. The gracilis muscle was harvested. The anterior tibial artery and both accompanying veins were dissected in the leg, preparing them for anastomosis to the gracilis muscle pedicle. **c.** The gracilis muscle was sutured into the edges of the wound. **d.** A meshed, split-thickness skin graft was stapled over the muscle. The entire procedure took 2.5 hours. **e** and **f.** In the final result, good soft-tissue cover has been achieved. The muscle has completely flattened out and profiles evenly with the surrounding tissues after approximately 6 months.

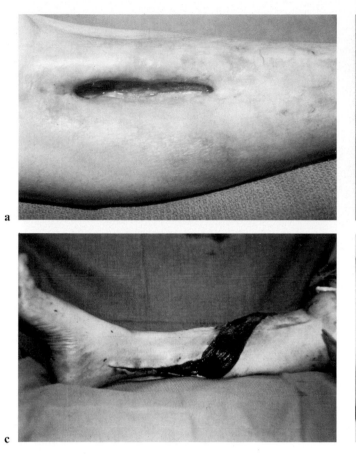

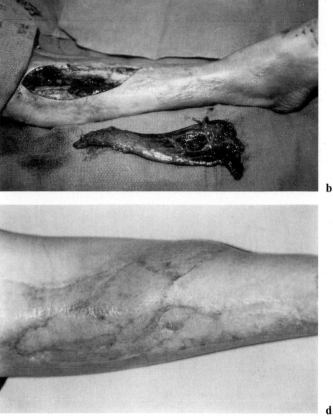

Fig. 1-10. a. A 46-year-old woman had had chronic osteomyelitis since being injured in a car accident 20 years earlier. The affected area, a wound located on the proximal lateral aspect of the leg, had been debrided many times but continued to drain, was inflamed, and had poor soft-tissue cover. The choice of recipient vessels was either the anterior tibial artery distal to the lesion, used in retrograde fashion, or the posterior tibial artery, which would require that the muscle course over the crest of the tibia. This latter option was chosen because of scarring around the anterior tibial vessel. (One of the most common causes of vascular problems following transplantation is the use of a vessel in the zone of injury.) **b.** Thorough debridement of the wound involved removing both soft tissue and bone. A local muscle pedicle flap was considered, but following appropriate debridement, it would probably not contour and fill all the dead space as completely as would a microvascular transplant. The gracilis muscle is shown ready to be placed in the defect. **c.** The microvascular transplant was connected end-to-side to the posterior tibial artery, and both gracilis veins were anastomosed to the venae comitantes. **d.** The transplant was covered with a split-thickness skin graft. Six months later excellent contour and adequate, well-vascularized soft-tissue cover was the result.

1.2.1.2 Traumatic Wounds – Chronic Stage, Wounds Surrounded by Irradiated Tissue, Osteomyelitis, and Infected Nonunions (Gordon and Chiu 1988, Mathes et al. 1982, May et al. 1984, Weiland et al. 1984).

In patients with *chronic osteomyelitis*, muscle tissue cover after debridement can usually control infection and reduce or eliminate drainage and other symptoms (Figs. 1-9 and 1-10). Muscle tissue holds up well when used to cover a variety of infected bone and soft-tissue wounds (Figs. 1-11 and 1-12). In wounds that have been previously infected, appropriate debridement is the cornerstone of treatment. Thorough debridement can be done with confidence, knowing that the resultant defect can be effectively covered with a muscle transplant (Figs. 3-3 and 3-5). To achieve a clean wound, several visits to the operating room may be required. Quantitative bacterial counts are valuable in establishing when wound cover should be performed. When that time has come, the muscle of appropriate size to cover the defect can then be selected (Fig. 1-13). Whereas *irradiated wounds* will often not heal, muscle transplants can introduce additional blood supply and effectively enable healing. Care must be taken to debride the wound adequately and place the vascular anastomoses beyond the irradiated region (Fig. 1-14).

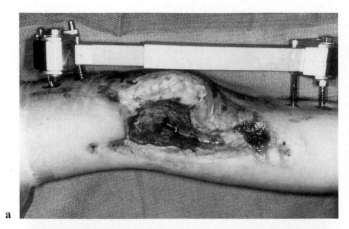

a

b

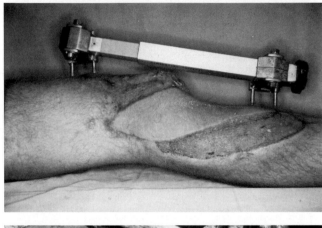

c

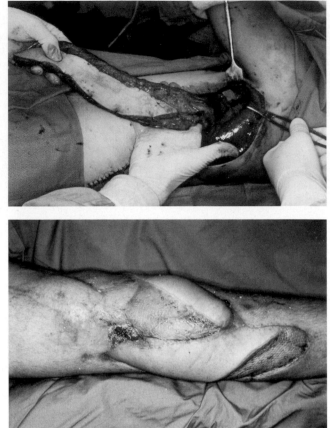

d

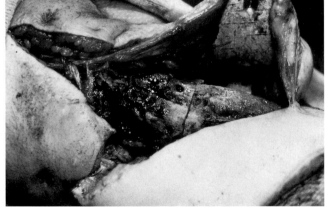

e

Fig. 1-11. a. An 18-year-old boy had an infected wound and osteomyelitis with inadequate soft-tissue cover involving the entire knee region. An external fixator with half-pins placed medially was used to stabilize the bones so that the anterior tibial vessels could be used distally on the lateral side of the leg. **b.** A latissimus dorsi musculocutaneous transplant was harvested from the left chest, and the pedicle was dissected. **c.** The latissimus dorsi flap covered the lateral defect, but anterior cover remained poor for any subsequent reconstruction. **d.** A second latissimus dorsi musculocutaneous transplant was used to provide good cover anteriorly. **e.** The cover was adequate for subsequent knee fusion using an external fixator. After osseous healing, no further drainage occurred despite the fact that the bone appeared infected at surgery. Both bone and soft tissues have remained healed and 2 years later the patient is fully weight bearing.

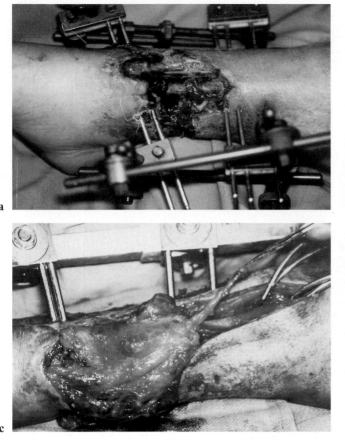
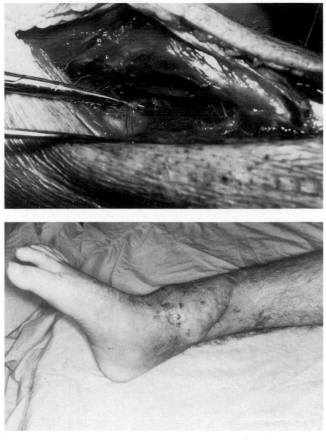

Fig. 1-12. a. This 22-year-old man suffered injuries in a motorcycle accident. This 1-month-old infected wound was too small for a latissimus dorsi muscle transplant unless only a small portion of the muscle were to be harvested. The defect was too wide for a gracilis transplant, but the lowest slips of the serratus anterior could be shaped to fit it well. **b.** In dissecting down to the recipient anterior tibial vessels, small vessels could be seen coursing between the tibialis anterior and extensor hallucis longus. These vessels easily led to the anterior tibial neurovascular bundle. **c.** The serratus anterior was harvested and fit the shape of the debrided wound. The muscle was sutured to the wound margins and the vessels were anastomosed. The muscle was covered with a split-thickness skin graft. **d.** The healed wound approximately 3 months later.

1.2.1.3 Exposed Metal (Plates, Prostheses) and Vital Anatomic Structures

A microvascular muscle transplant has the ability to cover foreign material because of its excellent vascularity and ability to closely contour the wound surface. Once again, meticulous debridement is essential (Figs. 1-15 and 1-28).

1.2.1.4 Contour Defects and Dead Space

Muscle tissue is excellent for filling the dead space of large wounds, especially those resulting from the loss of muscle or bone, or from debridement for infection (Fig. 1-16). Large cavities may also result from the removal of infected total joint prostheses where repeated infection has made salvage of the prosthesis impossible, or from tumor extirpation. In these situations, edema, fibrosis, and irradiated tissue frequently make local flaps unwise (Fig. 1-17). In general, excellent contour can be restored. Such defects can be covered with musculocutaneous transplants, or else the muscle tissue can be used alone and then covered with a split-thickness skin graft. The choice depends on the bulk needed to fill the defect and cover the wound.

1.2.1.5 Heel Wounds (Sec. 6.1.4)

Severe heel wounds can be covered with muscle tissue. The ultimate contour will usually be good, but care must be taken to choose a muscle of appropriate size. A musculocutaneous transplant is used for cutaneous cover over the weight-bearing region (Figs. 1-18 and 1-19). Although the latissimus dorsi is used most frequently for this purpose, the gracilis can be used as a musculocutaneous transplant. The cutaneous portion must be kept over the muscle and positioned in its proximal half (Fig. 1-20). For very extensive wounds with a large tissue defect, the tensor fasciae latae should be used. This muscle is particularly useful for heel wounds because the lateral femoral cutaneous nerve can be sutured to a nerve in the recipient area, restoring sensory return in the transplant (Fig. 1-21).

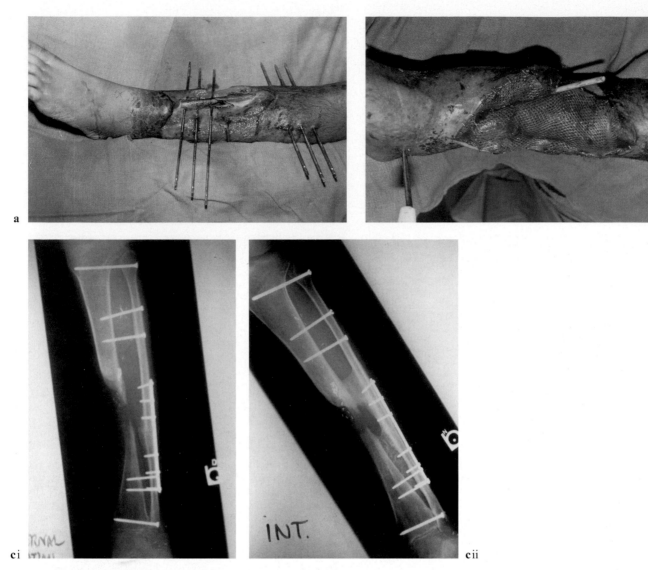

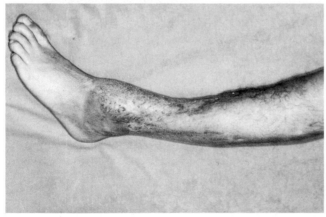

Fig. 1-13. a. An 18-year-old boy developed an infected leg wound 3 months after sustaining an open fracture of the tibia and fibula in a motorcycle accident. The necrotic bone and purulent drainage are seen. **b.** The external fixator was replaced so that the half-pins stood away from the wound. The wound was debrided and a latissimus dorsi muscle transplant was used for cover. **c.** Six months later the wound was entirely healed, allowing further osseous reconstruction. Because of the severity of the initial *Pseudomonas* infection, obtaining fibular healing with a plate (i) followed by a proximal and distal tibiofibular synostosis (ii) was decided upon. With this approach, the previously infected region was avoided during the subsequent bone grafting. (Courtesy of Dr. Floyd Jergesen, San Francisco, who performed the tibiofibular synostosis.) **d.** Three years later, the patient was fully weight bearing without difficulty and walked with a slight limp. Radiography showed a solid proximal and distal tibiofibular synostosis.

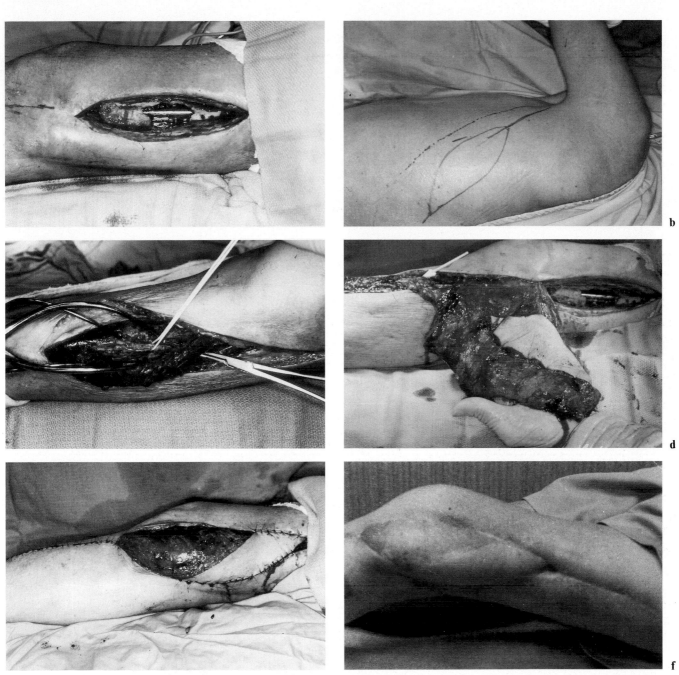

Fig. 1-14. a. Following the removal of a low-grade sarcoma, this intramedullary rod was exposed. An irradiated wound on the lateral aspect of the thigh was complicated by chronic infection. After debridement, a transplant was needed that would fill the dead space and introduce well-vascularized tissue. **b.** A latissimus dorsi musculocutaneous transplant was therefore planned to fill the defect and cover the wound. **c.** In the leg, the anterior tibial vessels were dissected (*in the vessel loop*), divided distally, and "swung" back under the tibialis anterior to be used as the donor vessels on the lateral aspect of the knee. **d.** The arrow indicates the location of the vascular anastomoses; the muscle is ready to be set into the defect. **e.** The muscle and skin provided excellent cover. A skin graft was used to cover the part of the muscle still exposed. **f.** The final result. The patient continues to use a cane, although the bone healed spontaneously on the medial aspect.

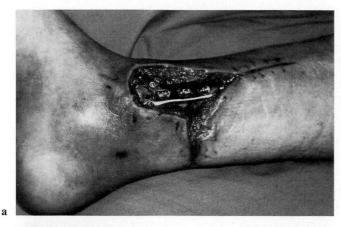

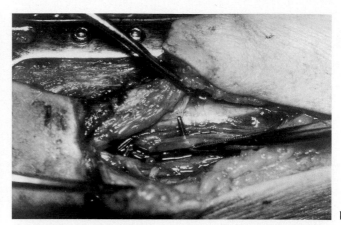

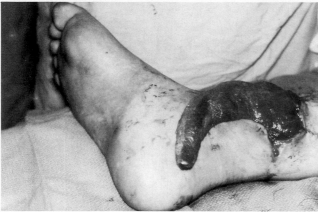

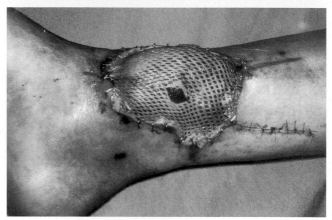

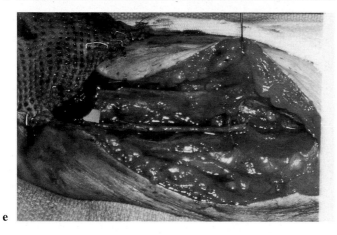

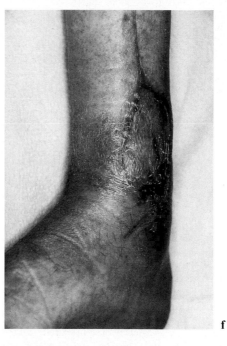

Fig. 1-15. a. A 60-year-old man sustained a comminuted fracture of the ankle requiring this plate. The crush injury caused the wound to break down. b. The posterior tibial vessels were dissected and the wound was meticulously cleaned and debrided. A close-up of these vessels is seen here. c. This wound was thought to be of ideal size and shape for a gracilis transplant, although the serratus anterior would also have fitted well. The gracilis muscle was loosely set into the defect while the vascular anastomoses were performed. d. The muscle was trimmed distally, set into the defect, and then covered with a split-thickness skin graft. e. Although it was felt that good vascularity was present initially, arterial thrombosis occurred approximately 3 hours later and an 8-cm vein graft was used to anastomose to the posterior tibial vessels more proximally in the leg. The initial repair was probably done with damaged vessels in the zone of injury. f. Excellent soft-tissue cover could be seen 4 months later.

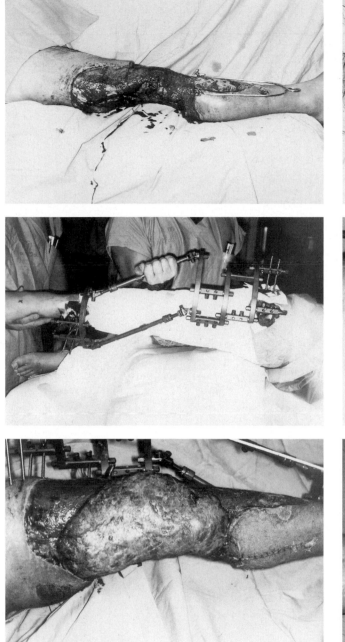

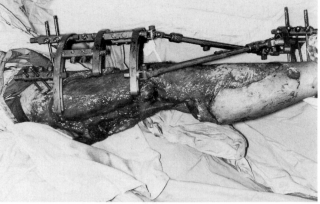

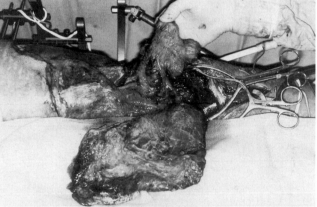

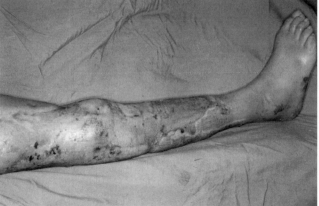

a

b

c

d

e

f

Fig. 1-16. a. This patient was a pedestrian when hit by a car. He sustained a supracondylar fracture with an open knee joint and this extensive amount of dead space and contour defect. The wound was circumferential, extending around the entire extremity. *Pseudomonas* and *Enterobacter* were found when the wound was cultured 10 days after the injury. **b.** An external fixation device with half-pins was placed which allowed access to the anterior tibial and posterior tibial vessels distal to the wound. The pins were placed in the skin so as not to interfere with subsequent muscle placement. (The external fixator must be placed to allow appropriate exposure of the entire wound and vessels. Familiarity with a versatile fixation device is essential.) Two radical debridement procedures were performed to ensure that the wound was as clean as possible and all necrotic material had been removed. **c.** This external fixator provided stability for the bones in all planes and simplified the six hourly dressing changes. **d.** The posterior aspect of the knee is shown. A combined latissimus dorsi-serratus anterior transplant was planned. The serratus anterior was used to fill the dead space and cover the knee joint and fracture, while the latissimus dorsi provided overlying soft-tissue cover. Suction-irrigation tubes were placed in the medial aspect of the knee and remained there until culture results from the tubes were negative, which was about 7 days later. **e.** The latissimus transplant is seen overlying the area of the defect and the serratus muscle. The vessels were anastomosed to the posterior tibial vessels, distal to the injury. **f.** The defect was covered with a split-thickness skin graft, and healing was achieved within 2 weeks. The leg is seen here 3 months later. A knee fusion performed 4 months after injury involved elevating the transplant and placing bone graft. A solid fusion was obtained.

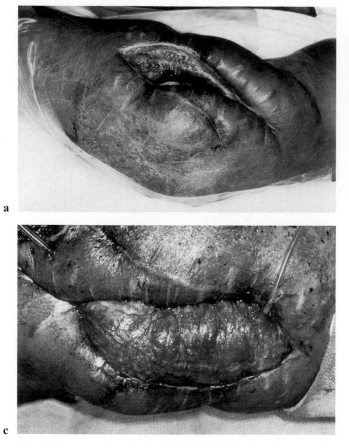

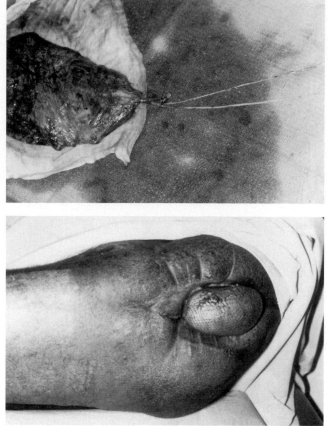

Fig. 1-17. a. A 28-year-old patient with sickle cell disease was left with this large infected wound extending down to the acetabulum and proximal femur following removal of an infected total hip prosthesis. After four attempts at total hip replacement, a Girdlestone procedure was decided upon. Several local flaps had failed, resulting in extensive fibrosis around the hip region. Because of the sickle cell disease, the patient was given an exchange transfusion preoperatively. **b.** A latissimus dorsi muscle transplant was chosen to fill this extensive defect. Because of the extremely poor surrounding tissues, 18-cm vein grafts were harvested; on a separate table in the operating room, these vein grafts were anastomosed to the thoracodorsal artery and vein prior to insertion of the muscle into the defect. The inferior epigastric vessels were used as the recipient vessels. **c.** The latissimus dorsi can be seen filling the defect. Suction and irrigation tubes were placed in the depths of the wound and left there for approximately 5 days. **d.** The transplant was covered with a split-thickness skin graft, and it healed without subsequent problems. At the 4-year follow-up examination, no problems or recurrent infection had been experienced, and the patient was able to fully bear weight with a limp following the Girdlestone procedure.

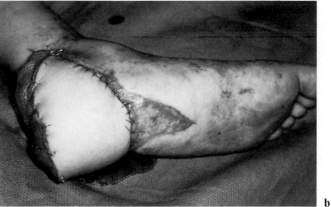

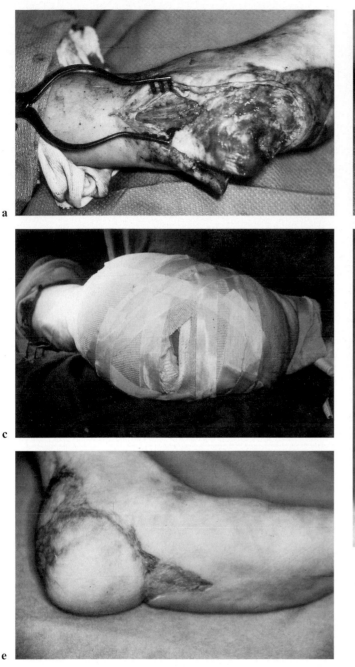

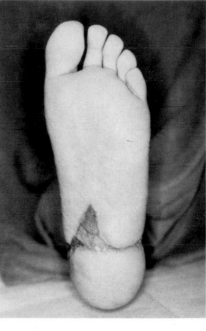

Fig. 1-18. a. A 22-year-old sailor sustained an avulsive injury to the heel which subsequently became infected. The wound was debrided and the posterior tibial artery and accompanying veins were dissected as recipient vessels. **b.** A latissimus dorsi musculocutaneous transplant was used, with the muscle filling the dead space and the cutaneous portion providing cover over the heel. **c.** A window through all levels of the dressing allowed the vascularity of the transplant to be monitored postoperatively. **d** and **e.** One year later the transplant had atrophied considerably, providing good contour. The patient is able to walk normally with special footwear. (I thank Charlotte Alexander, M.D., Oak Knoll Naval Hospital, who was the cosurgeon on this procedure.)

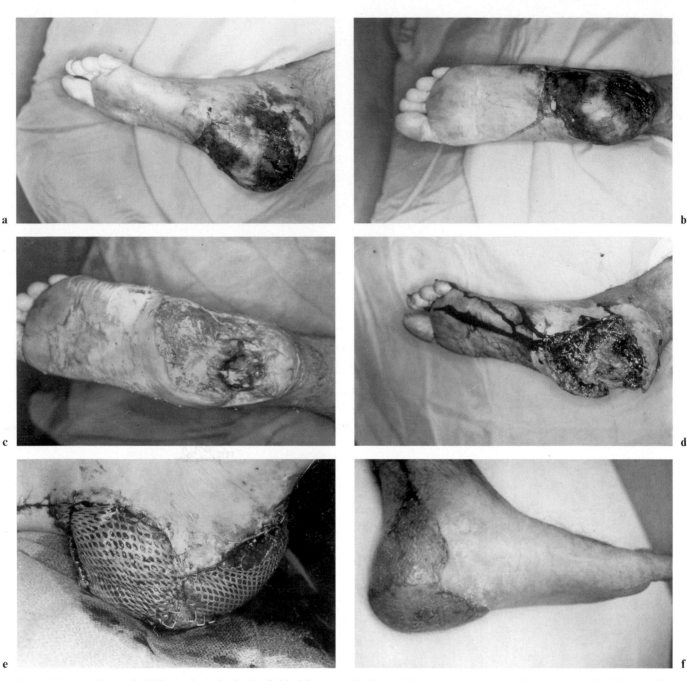

Fig. 1-19. a and **b.** A forklift crushed the heel of this laborer and also caused an underlying fracture of the calcaneus. The heel initially appeared viable but became necrotic 10 days later. (Necrosis of the heel only becomes evident after 7–10 days.) **c** and **d**. Debridement of the necrotic tissue left an extensive defect in the weight-bearing portion of the heel. **e**. The defect was covered with a latissimus dorsi musculocutaneous transplant. The cutaneous part was used over the heel, and the rest of the muscle was covered with a split-thickness skin graft. **f.** The contour is good, and the split-thickness skin graft on the weight-bearing part of the sole can be removed as the muscle atrophies. The patient is able to fully bear weight and walk without a limp, but occasionally has trouble with breakdown that requires him to stay off his heel. He found it necessary to change to a sedentary occupation.

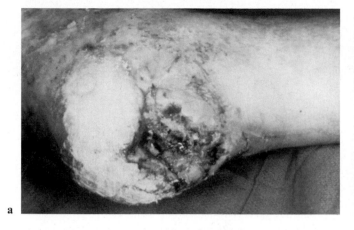

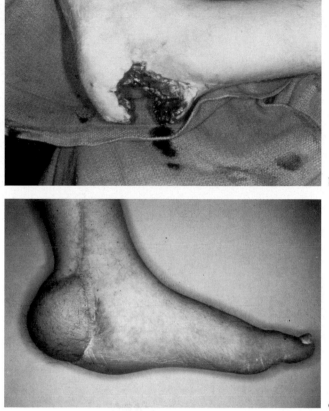

Fig. 1-20. a. A grossly infected heel 4 months after a gunshot wound. **b.** The condition of the wound necessitated radical debridement back to bleeding tissue to remove all infected and necrotic matter. **c.** A gracilis musculocutaneous transplant was used. The muscle itself filled the defect, with the cutaneous portion used for a serviceable heel surface. (Because the cutaneous portion must be placed proximally and the vascularity is not entirely reliable, this transplant is rarely used.)

1.2.1.6 Amputation Stumps (Sec. 6.1.6)

Short *below-knee or below-elbow amputation stumps* can be covered with a muscle or musculocutaneous transplant. Such cover obviates the need to shorten a stump that is already too short. It is very important to save the knee or elbow joint and make a below-elbow or below-knee prosthesis possible (Fig. 1-22).

1.2.1.7 Complex Wounds

When wounds involve the loss of several different tissues, such as muscle, bone, and nerve, a decision must be made as to whether extremity salvage is wise. This decision partly depends on whether a muscle transplant can achieve vascularized cover without the complication of infection. Extremity salvage may not be appropriate if there is loss of bone and muscle in the presence of infection, especially with gram-negative organisms. For this reason, in such complex wounds, I prefer to treat the problem in stages. First, muscle tissue is used to achieve a healed wound. If no infection is present, vascularized or conventional bone grafting is done 2–3

months later (Chapter 3). Attempting to reconstruct the entire area with simultaneous bone and muscle transplantation is risky and will often fail because of infection and poor healing.

1.2.1.8 Wounds in High-Risk Patients

Whereas conventional solutions are often doomed to failure if not impossible, muscle transplantation can frequently salvage an extremity in "high-risk" clinical situations. To do so, great care in preoperative planning is essential. Some patients who could be considered as high risk are those who are morbidly obese (Fig. 1-23), diabetic, and those who have sickle cell disease (Fig. 1-17). Also in this category are the elderly (Fig. 2-3), the infirm, and those who have a serious illness but need rapid and effective cover to allow them more mobility. None of these factors contraindicate microvascular procedures. Careful judgement is important because major surgery may be too risky. At times, however, microsurgical alternatives are the simplest and best method of mobilizing such patients.

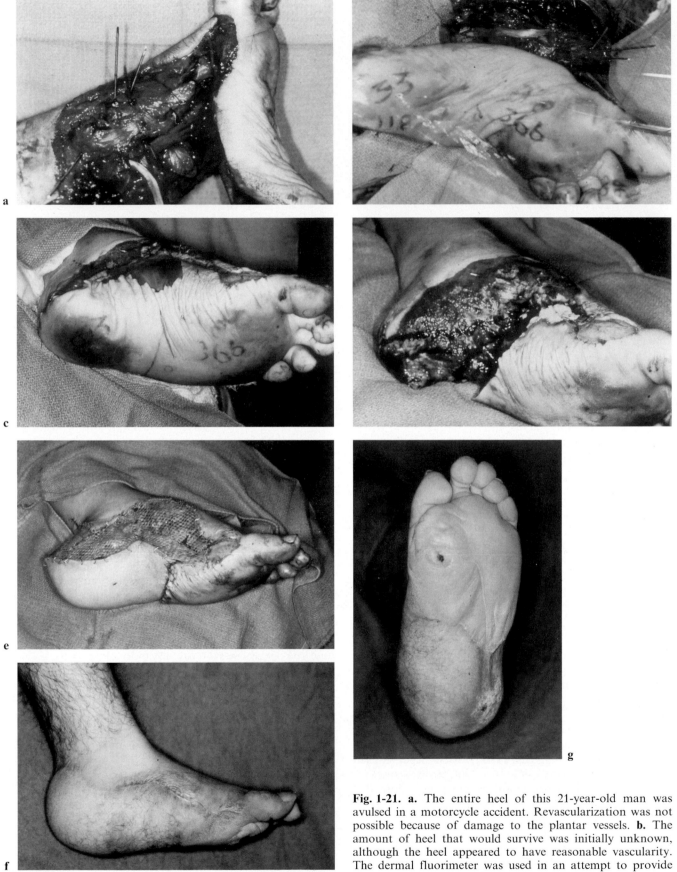

Fig. 1-21. a. The entire heel of this 21-year-old man was avulsed in a motorcycle accident. Revascularization was not possible because of damage to the plantar vessels. **b.** The amount of heel that would survive was initially unknown, although the heel appeared to have reasonable vascularity. The dermal fluorimeter was used in an attempt to provide

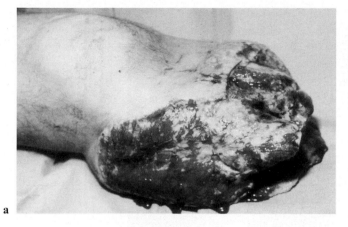

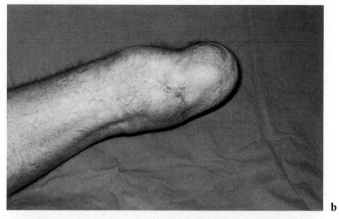

a

b

Fig. 1-22. a. This 38-year-old man was involved in a logging accident in which his right leg was crushed and amputated below the knee. The short below-knee bone stump had a sagittal fracture without extension into the knee, and the soft tissues were severely crushed. After thorough debridement, a latissimus dorsi musculocutaneous transplant was used to cover the amputation stump. Because the patient had severe injuries to his other leg, salvage of the knee joint was particularly desirable. **b** and **c.** Good cover was achieved but the flap became redundant and there was breakdown over the split-thickness skin-grafted portion. Two debulking procedures were necessary, and a tissue expander was used to bring both the medial and lateral skin over the amputation stump so that it was covered almost entirely with full-thickness skin. The patient regained 90° of knee motion and is able to wear a below-knee prosthesis without difficulty or limp.

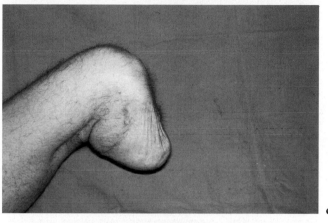

c

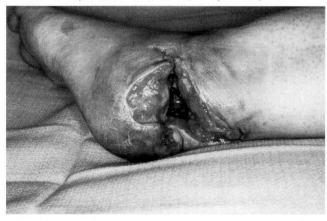

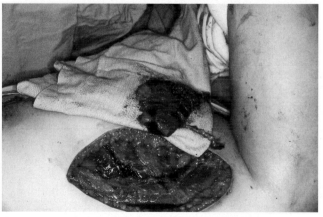

a

b

Fig. 1-23. a. A morbidly obese teenager had fractured femurs and other injuries after a car accident. This chronically infected wound of the ankle with calcaneal osteomyelitis needed debridement and filling of the defect with good vascularized tissue. Although it was not large, the wound was deep and would not heal. (The serratus anterior muscle is ideal for this type of problem.) **b.** The serratus anterior was harvested. Only the lowest two digitations were removed. Note the long vascular pedicle (Continued.).

◁

a prognosis. The readings before and after intravenous injection of 1 cc of fluorescein are shown. **c.** The flap was loosely sutured back into position. After approximately 8 days, the amount of necrosis in the heel could be assessed (see also Fig. 1-33). **d.** The necrotic skin was resected, leaving an extensive defect. **e.** A tensor fasciae latae musculocutaneous transplant was used to fill the defect and provide cutaneous cover. (It is important to place this transplant longitudinally if at all possible when used in the heel. If not, it will be bulky and contour will be poor.) Part of the transplant on the medial aspect of the foot was covered with a split-thickness skin graft. **f** and **g.** After debulking, the heel had good contour and cover. This patient was subsequently able to pass the mile run and other tests required to become a fire fighter. In a 4-year period, the patient experienced one episode of temporary breakdown, but the area healed spontaneously.

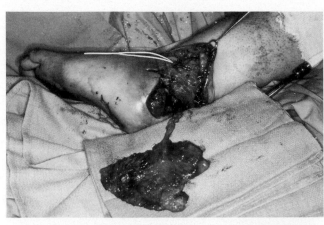

ci

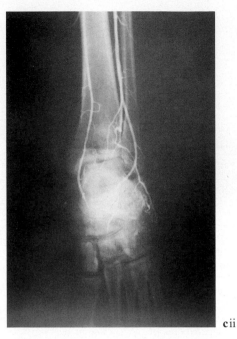

cii

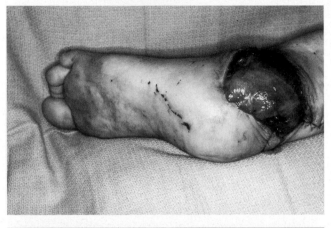

d

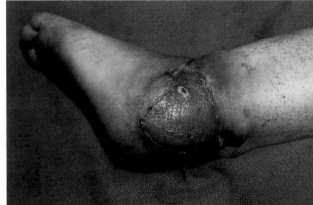

e

Fig. 1-23. c. (i) The wound was debrided and the flap is seen ready to be placed in the defect. (ii) The anterior tibial artery, found originating from the fibular side in this patient (*in the vessel loop*), was dissected as a donor vessel (Plate 4-III). **d.** The muscle was set into the defect, filling its depths. **e.** The transplant 1 month later. It takes approximately 6–12 months for the muscle to atrophy and profile evenly with the surrounding skin.

1.2.2 Functional Muscle Transplantation
(Manktelow and McKee 1979, O'Brien et al. 1982)

The need for functional muscle transplantation arises where massive *muscle loss* has occurred, such as after Volkmann's ischemia or a crush, blast, or avulsive injury. This procedure is indicated only if no other tendon transfers are possible. Muscle transplantation cannot be used after severe nerve injuries (such as brachial plexus avulsions), as no recipient nerve will be available. The *finger flexors* are the muscle group most fre-

quently substituted, but reconstruction of the *finger extensors* may occasionally be indicated using a functional muscle transplant. Following this procedure, the muscle can be expected to lose 30–50% of its original strength (Terzis et al. 1978), but enough strength and excursion will remain for functional range of motion of the fingers with useful pinch and grip. *Elbow flexion* is usually restored with the pectoralis major, latissimus dorsi, or forearm flexors. If none of these are available and a recipient nerve is present, a microvascular muscle transplant may then be used. Functional muscle transplanta-

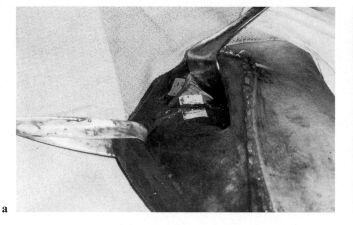

a

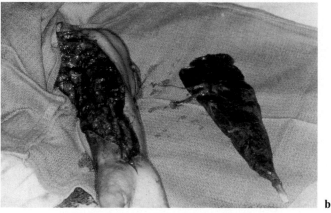

b

Fig. 1-24. a. The gracilis muscle has been dissected (*shown in the Penrose drain*). The adductor longus muscle is being retracted, and the vascular pedicle (*under the blue background*) can be seen coursing under this muscle to supply the gracilis. A pedicle measuring 7 cm has been dissected. The anterior branch of the obturator nerve (*under the yellow background*) superficial to the adductor brevis can be seen joining the vascular pedicle at the neurovascular hilus. **b.** The muscle has been removed and the proximal and distal tendons divided. The vascular and nerve pedicles are seen entering the muscle.

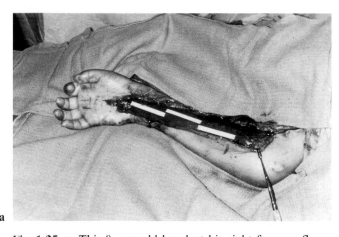

a

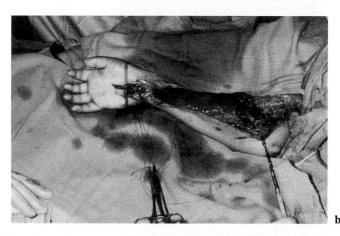

b

Fig. 1-25. a. This 8-year-old boy lost his right forearm flexor muscles after sustaining a supracondylar fracture and Volkmann's ischemia. The gracilis muscle can be seen in position. The proximal tendon (taken from the pubis) was attached to the medial epicondyle, and the distal tendon was attached to the flexor digitorum profundus tendons at the wrist. Next, the vasculature was restored, and the obturator nerve (supplying the gracilis) was sutured to the anterior interosseous nerve. **b.** It is important that the muscle fibers enjoy the same resting length in the transplant site as they did in the donor site. To ensure this, sutures or other markers should be placed every 5 cm along the muscle prior to dividing either of the tendons in the thigh. These markers should remain the same distance apart after the muscle has been sutured proximally and distally in the forearm. If adequate skin is present, the muscle is buried, but it will function just as well if covered with a split-thickness skin graft.

tion for *lower-extremity problems* has not been used with success. The excursion, size, and single nerve supply of the *gracilis* make this muscle useful as a substitute for long finger flexors and other muscles (Fig. 1-24). However, functional muscle transplantation depends on the presence of a recipient motor nerve. In the forearm, the anterior interosseous is the nerve most commonly used for this purpose (Fig. 1-25), but in some circumstances the motor fascicles of the ulnar nerve may be used.

Other muscles such as the latissimus dorsi and pectoralis major have also occasionally been used as functional muscle transplants. These are strong muscles but with less excursion than the gracilis. In rare circumstances, the slips of the serratus anterior can be used for both cover and restoring thumb opposition; in this situation, the recipient motor nerve used is the recurrent branch of the median nerve, which is repaired to the fascicles of the long thoracic nerve supplying the lowest digitations of the muscle (Fig. 4-8) (Gordon et al. 1984).

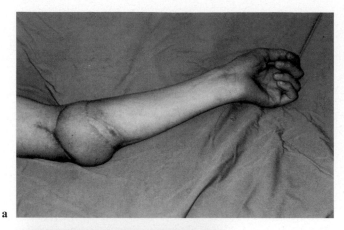

a

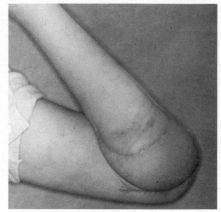

b

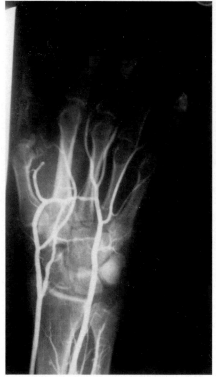

c

Fig. 1-26. a and b. A latissimus dorsi transplant was used in this patient to cover an extensive medial elbow wound that involved loss of the medial collateral ligament and part of the elbow joint. The cutaneous portion of the transplant was used to cover the region of the elbow crease to prevent later breakdown. Subsequent nerve grafting was done under this flap. c. The arteriogram showed the presence of *separate* radial and ulnar arterial supplies to the hand. For this reason, the radial artery could not be used in retrograde fashion as a recipient artery (see Chapter 7).

1.3 Choice of Muscle Transplant

The *pedicle* of any reliable muscle transplant must have a constant anatomic location and be the dominant vascular supply to the muscle (Mathes and Nahai 1981). Transplantation is considerably easier if the length and diameter of the pedicle is large; preferably, it should average 2 mm in external diameter and be long enough to allow positioning of the anastomosis away from the zone of injury. Each of the four muscle transplants described in this chapter have these features. The dimensions of the vessels supplying these flaps are given in Table 1-1.

The latissimus pedicle consists of the thoracodorsal artery and a single large and patulous vena comitans. The latissimus dorsi is composed of a large amount

of muscle tissue, and when the artery is anastomosed to a major vessel in the lower extremity, the inflow and outflow are great. The somewhat sclerotic veins of the lower extremity may not dilate sufficiently to

Table 1-1. Vessel parameters of various muscle transplants.

Transplant	Length (cm)	Artery diameter (mm)	Vein diameter (mm)
Latissimus dorsi	6	2	2.0–2.5 (one only)
Gracilis	5	1.5	1.0–1.5 (two veins)
Serratus anterior	10	2	2.0–2.5 (one only)
Tensor fasciae latae	4	2	1.5–2.0 (two veins)

Fig. 1-27. a. The donor site following excision of the *gracilis transplant* is inconspicuous and situated on the medial aspect of the thigh. **b.** (i) A contour defect may result at the *latissimus dorsi donor site* in muscular individuals, but it is in a fairly inconspicuous location. (ii) The donor site of the *serratus anterior* is similar to that of the latissimus dorsi, but there is no contour defect. A mild amount of scapular winging can occur but is not functionally significant. **c.** The donor site following excision of the *tensor fasciae latae transplant* can usually be closed primarily with an excellent cosmetic result. If it is too wide, split-thickness skin grafting is required and the appearance is poor because of the contour defect.

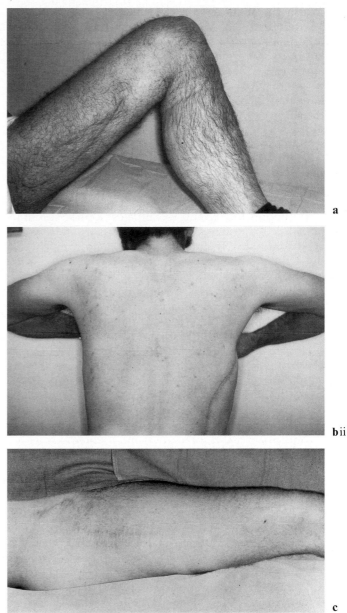

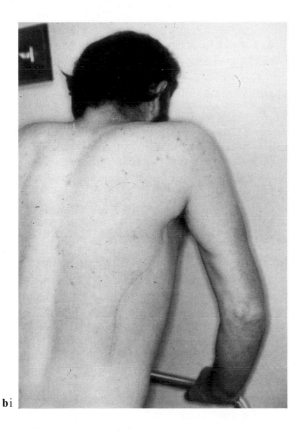

allow enough venous drainage, especially if there has been some venous disease; if that is the case, a smaller muscle transplant should be chosen if possible. Also in patients with chronic venous disease, the venae comitantes may have thinner, more dilatable walls, which would make them better recipient veins than those in the saphenous system. The serratus anterior pedicle is usually dissected proximal to the origin of the thoracodorsal vessels to provide a very long pedicle. The pedicle can also be used closer to the muscle where it consists of the serratus branch of the thoracodorsal vessel. The gracilis and tensor fasciae latae pedicles contain one artery and two venae comitantes (Table 1-1).

Variable size and shape are among the greatest virtues of muscle transplantation (Fig. 1-1). The appropriate size muscle can be chosen and then contoured to the form of the defect being treated. Muscle size varies with the stature of the individual. For example, older female patients have small gracilis muscles. In an average individual, the gracilis is approximately 5×20 cm; the latissimus dorsi, 15×25–30 cm; the serratus, 2×8 cm for each digitation (a total of three digitations may be used); and the tensor fasciae latae, 8×25 cm.

When choosing the size of transplant needed, one should take into account (1) that further debridement may be required at the time of surgery; (2) the location of the vascular anastomosis, which must be outside the zone of injury; and (3) the volume of dead space to be filled. One should choose a muscle slightly larger than the defect so that the muscle can be trimmed to fit exactly. Wounds in the distal tibia and other such anatomic sites that are extremely difficult to cover by other methods can be effectively treated by microvascular muscle transplantation. A small part of the serratus anterior can be used for a small defect, while defects of intermediate size can be covered with the gracilis. Even the largest of defects involving the majority of the surface of the leg can be covered with the latissimus dorsi, which, as mentioned, can be combined with the serratus anterior.

A muscle can be transplanted along with its overlying skin as a *musculocutaneous transplant*, or it can be used alone and then covered with a *split-thickness skin graft* (Gordon et al. 1984, Nahai and Mathes 1984). This latter option has several advantages. Donor site morbidity is reduced because the donor wound can be closed primarily without tension. At the recipient site the transplant is less bulky, so the contour is often better. The muscle can be flipped over to use the superficial surface deep; this is sometimes more convenient for performing the vascular anastomosis. Through-and-through defects can be closed, filling the dead space and covering both sides with a split-thickness skin graft (Fig. 3-3). In the region of the antecubital fossa, popliteal fossa, or other skin creases, muscle tissue covered with a skin graft tends to break down, so a musculocutaneous transplant is preferable (Fig. 1-26), with the cutaneous portion positioned over the skin crease.

Muscles tend to *atrophy* considerably (especially if the motor nerve is not repaired) and become extensively replaced by fibrous tissue. Initially the contour tends to be too bulky, but it "settles down" and becomes flat over the next 6 to 12 months. The *skin grafts* placed directly on muscle tissue tend to "take" excellently, and nearly 100% can be expected to be successful. These grafts, when taken from the lateral thigh, usually develop an excellent color match when used in the extremities; one exception is in dark-skinned individuals when these grafts are used in the palm.

The *donor sites* of these muscle and musculocutaneous transplants can always be closed primarily, except for that of the tensor fasciae latae; this transplant should be kept quite narrow to allow primary closure (Fig. 1-27). If that is not possible, skin grafting, which is quite unsightly, will be required. At a later date, a tissue expander can be used so that the skin graft can be removed (Sec. 1.6.2.2).

The *gracilis* is entirely expendable, as the rest of the adductor muscle group takes over its function. The gracilis incision is made on the medial aspect of the thigh and is well concealed.

Removal of the *latissimus dorsi* produces a contour defect in muscular individuals, but one that is not very noticeable. The scar on the lateral chest is inconspicuous. Except in some avid athletes, removal of the latissimus dorsi is unlikely to result in any noticeable weak-

ness, and even patients who swim regularly have not experienced a significant problem.

The *serratus anterior* scar is inconspicuous and similar to that of the latissimus dorsi. The lowest digitations are removed, retaining the integrity of the nerve supply to the upper six digitations and, therefore, muscle function. There is usually a minor amount of scapular winging on very careful scrutiny, but experience has shown that patients have no symptoms following this transplant.

Following *tensor fasciae latae* transplantation, there is no detectable motor functional deficit, but the cosmetic problem can be substantial if skin grafting is needed.

1.4 Gracilis Muscle Transplantation
(Harii et al. 1976)

1.4.1 Anatomy (Plates 1-I and 1-II)

The gracilis is the most superficial of the adductor group of thigh muscles and is entirely expendable. It *arises* by a broad tendon along the entire length of the inferior pubic ramus. The muscle is broader proximally and then tapers as it passes distally to *insert* into the upper part of the shaft of the tibia as the pes anserinus, between the sartorius and semitendinosus tendons. The muscle is somewhat cylindrical in shape. Its size is quite variable and depends on the level of thigh muscle development. For this reason it is generally smaller in women.

The *vascularity* of the muscle is supplied by three pedicles: a proximal, major pedicle and two minor, distal ones. The *major pedicle* can adequately supply the entire muscle. This pedicle consists of an artery and paired venae comitantes. The artery rarely measures less than 1.5 mm in external diameter, but may be small in obese women with poorly developed thigh muscles. The pedicle enters the gracilis about 10 cm distal to the pubic tubercle (Mathes and Nahai 1979). It arises from the medial circumflex artery deep to the adductor longus muscle, and lies on the adductor magnus before entering the deep surface of the gracilis somewhat nearer its anterior than its posterior margin. It often divides into two branches – one ascending and one descending – before entering the gracilis. Pedicle length is 6-8 cm if taken back to the medial circumflex vessels. Along its course, it gives several branches to the adductor longus and other surrounding muscles.

The *obturator nerve* (L2–L4) exits the obturator foramen and divides into an *anterior* and a posterior branch which travel anterior and posterior to the adductor brevis muscle, respectively. The anterior branch then lies on the adductor magnus to join the vascular pedicle near its entry into the gracilis.

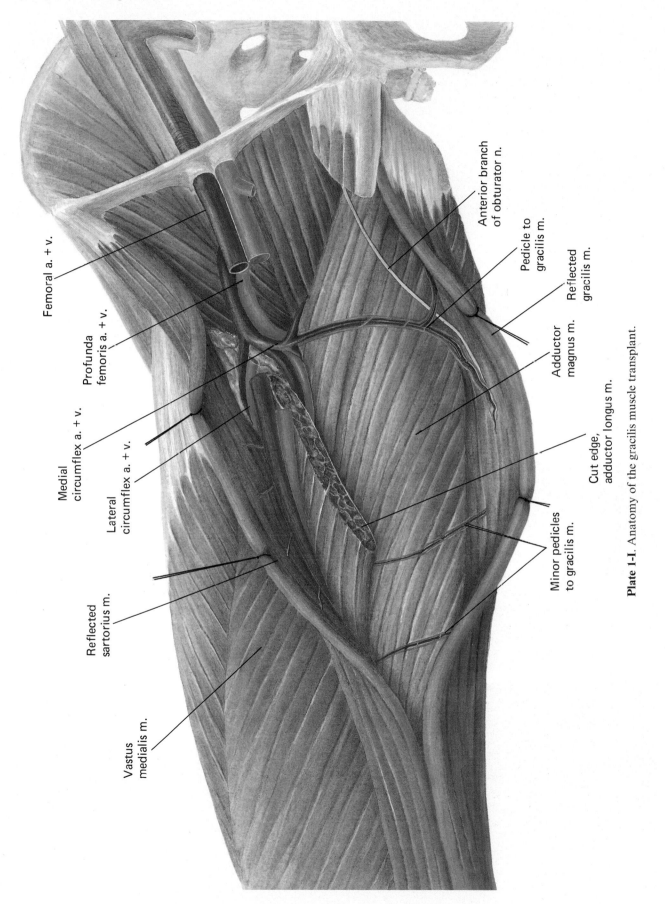

Femoral a. + v.

Profunda femoris a. + v.

Medial circumflex a. + v.

Lateral circumflex a. + v.

Reflected sartorius m.

Vastus medialis m.

Anterior branch of obturator n.

Pedicle to gracilis m.

Reflected gracilis m.

Adductor magnus m.

Cut edge, adductor longus m.

Minor pedicles to gracilis m.

Plate 1-I. Anatomy of the gracilis muscle transplant.

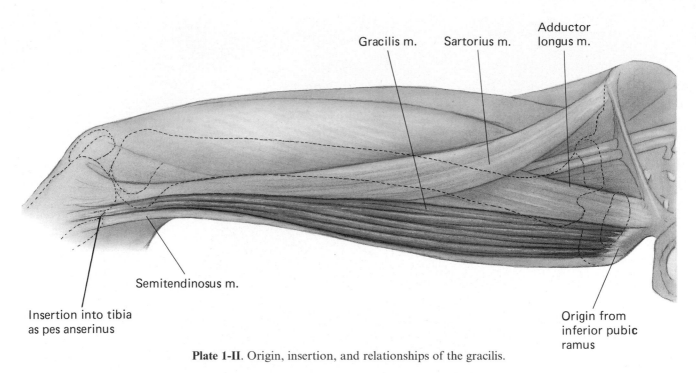

Gracilis m.   Sartorius m.   Adductor longus m.

Semitendinosus m.

Insertion into tibia as pes anserinus

Origin from inferior pubic ramus

Plate 1-II. Origin, insertion, and relationships of the gracilis.

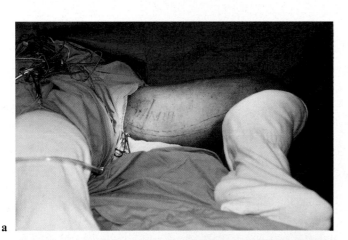

a

1.4.2 Surgical Technique
(Fig. 1-28; see also Fig. 1-15)

a. The position of the patient for dissection of the gracilis muscle is shown. The hip is abducted and externally rotated, and the knee is flexed, putting the gracilis muscle on stretch.

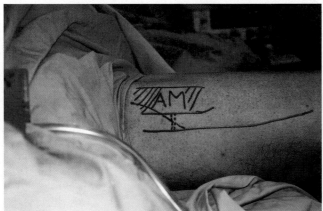

b

b. The proposed incision and relevant structures are outlined. The adductor longus muscle (AM) can be palpated as a firm band on the medial aspect of the thigh. The axis of the gracilis is parallel and 1–2 in. posterior to this band. (There is a tendency to make the incision too anterior.) The anticipated position of the vascular pedicle is marked approximately 10 cm from the pubic tubercle. The position of the anterior branch of the obturator nerve is also outlined.

c. The position of the gracilis muscle is identified, noting the direction of its fibers. The sartorius is more anterior, with fibers traveling proximally and laterally toward the anterior superior iliac spine. A Penrose drain is placed around the muscle distally. One of the two or three minor pedicles of the gracilis is shown here.

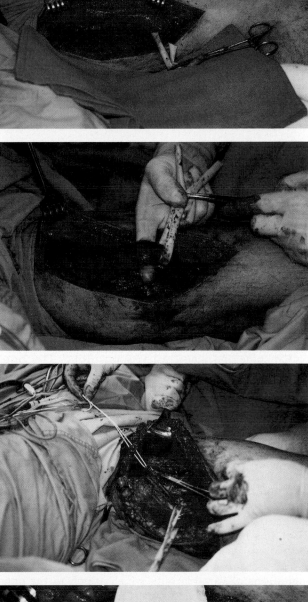

c

d. By lifting on the Penrose drain, the muscle is easily separated from the surrounding tissues by finger dissection, and the minor pedicles are divided.

d

e. As dissection proceeds to the proximal third of the muscle, the vascular pedicle is encountered in its reliable position entering the muscle laterally. In this dissection the vessel loop is around the obturator nerve, and the clamp is under the vascular pedicle as it passes deep to the adductor longus.

f. The pedicle is seen dissected. A large Richardson retractor is used to strongly retract the adductor longus muscle so that the pedicle can be dissected deep into the thigh; this provides a pedicle of 5 cm or longer. Small branches from the pedicle to the other adductor muscles are encountered which mostly travel anteriorly into the adductor longus. These branches are carefully ligated and divided to prevent troublesome bleeding as the pedicle is dissected. (Rather than "skeletonizing" the pedicle, it is easier to longitudinally incise the fascia over the adductor longus 1–2 mm away from the pedicle and let this fascia drop down toward the pedicle as increased pedicle length is dissected.)

It is not unusual for the pedicle to divide before reaching the anterior border of the gracilis. Care should therefore be taken to dissect both branches of the pedicle back to their common parent trunk. This pattern can usually be detected by noting the direction of the vessel's approach as it nears the muscle.

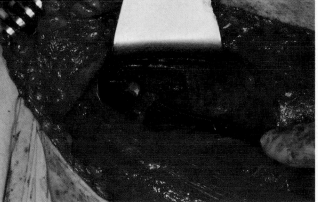

e

f

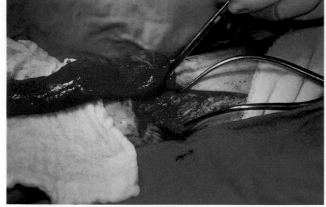

g

g. The proximal and distal tendons are divided, the pedicle is divided, and the muscle is transplanted to the recipient area. (It is important to have the recipient area completely dissected and ready for the transplant so that ischemia time is minimized.) The muscle is loosely sutured at a few points to avoid accidentally moving it during the vascular anastomoses.

1.5 Serratus Anterior and Latissimus Dorsi Muscle Transplantation

(Takayanagi and Tsukie 1982)

1.5.1 Anatomy (Plates 1-III to 1-V)

The *latissimus dorsi* is a broad, triangular muscle. It *originates* from the spinous processes of the lower six thoracic vertebrae and the posterior third of the iliac crest. Between these two attachments, it fuses with the thoracolumbar fascia, and can have muscular slips of origin from the lower three or four ribs. Its attachment to the spine and iliac crest is aponeurotic. This origin is the base of the triangle, and as the muscle passes to the apex at its insertion, it attaches to the inferior angle of the scapula. It has an elongated tendinous *insertion* into the intertubercular groove of the proximal humerus.

The latissimus dorsi is a medial rotator of the humerus, and extends the arm from the flexed position, as when swimming the crawl stroke. Its removal results in a contour defect in muscular individuals. The scar is inconspicuous but does have a tendency to spread. Surprisingly little functional deficit results from removal of this muscle, even in swimmers and other active individuals.

The *serratus anterior* muscle *arises* by eight or nine digitations of variable bulk which attach to the upper eight or nine ribs. The lowest four or five interdigitate with the slips of origin of the external oblique muscle, which pass distally. The muscle slips converge as they approach their *insertion*, passing deep to the scapula to insert into its entire medial border.

The serratus anterior keeps the scapula close to the thorax. It rotates the scapula in adduction and abduction of the arm. After removal of the lowest two or three digitations, there is very mild scapular winging but no significant functional deficit.

The *vascular supply* to both these muscles arises from the subscapular artery. This artery emanates from the axillary artery at the lower border of the subscapularis muscle. About 4 cm from its origin it divides into the circumflex scapular artery (Sec. 2.5.1) and the *thoracodorsal artery*. The thoracodorsal artery is accompanied by a single large vein. By ligating and dividing the branch to the latissimus dorsi, it can be used to vascularize the serratus anterior transplant. By ligating and dividing the branch to the serratus anterior, it vascularizes the latissimus transplant. If desired, both muscles can be transplanted simultaneously.

The thoracodorsal artery continues the general course of the subscapular artery, proceeding toward the latissimus dorsi, which it enters about 5 to 8 cm later. There, it divides into two branches running longitudinally. One travels within 2 to 3 cm of the anterior margin of the muscle, and the other runs just posterior to the midline of the muscle. The muscle can be split longitudinally between these two branches, maintaining adequate vascular supply to each (Fig. 1-30j). The latissimus dorsi is also supplied segmentally by minor pedicles from the intercostal and lumbar arteries which enter the deep surface of the posterior part of the muscle. The thoracodorsal artery has a single, patulous vena comitans.

Just before entering the latissimus dorsi, the thoracodorsal artery gives off a branch that passes onto the chest wall and runs on the *serratus anterior*. This artery travels longitudinally a few centimeters anterior to the lateral border of the scapula. The lateral thoracic artery also runs longitudinally on the serratus anterior but is more anterior, lying near where the muscle slips attach to the ribs anteriorly.

The *thoracodorsal nerve* (C7–C8), which serves the latissimus dorsi, is a branch of the posterior cord of the brachial plexus. It travels with the thoracodorsal artery.

The serratus anterior muscle is innervated by the *long thoracic nerve* (C–C7). This nerve arises from the roots of the brachial plexus in the neck, passes posterior to the plexus, and enters the axilla between the axillary artery and the serratus anterior. It then proceeds longitudinally down the muscle near the vascular pedicle. Its position may vary, but it is usually 1-2 cm anterior to the major vascular pedicle. Along its course, it sends small fascicles to each digitation as it crosses over them.

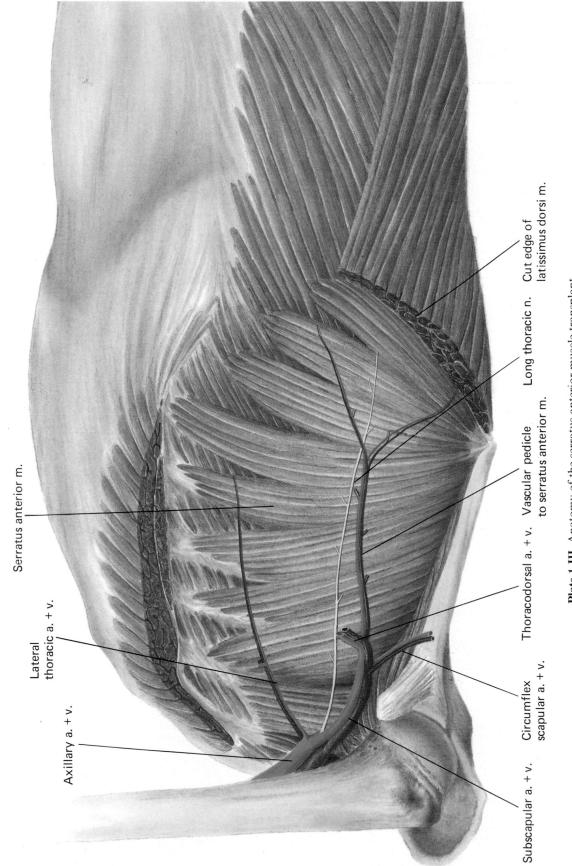

Serratus anterior m.

Lateral
thoracic a. + v.

Axillary a. + v.

Subscapular a. + v.

Circumflex
scapular a. + v.

Thoracodorsal a. + v.

Vascular pedicle
to serratus anterior m.

Long thoracic n.

Cut edge of
latissimus dorsi m.

Plate 1-III. Anatomy of the serratus anterior muscle transplant.

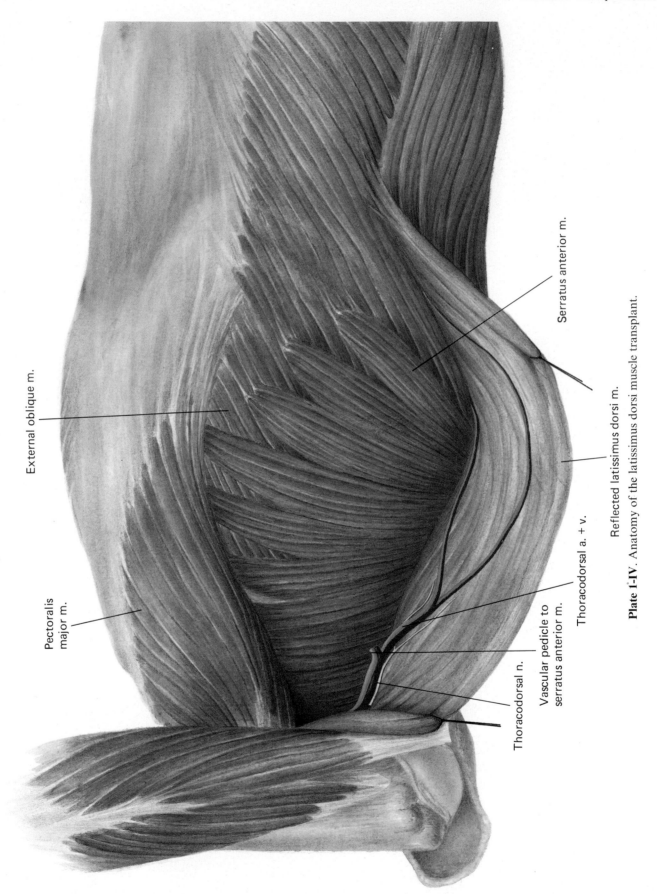

Serratus anterior m.

Reflected latissimus dorsi m.

External oblique m.

Thoracodorsal a. + v.

Pectoralis major m.

Thoracodorsal n.

Vascular pedicle to serratus anterior m.

Plate 1-IV. Anatomy of the latissimus dorsi muscle transplant.

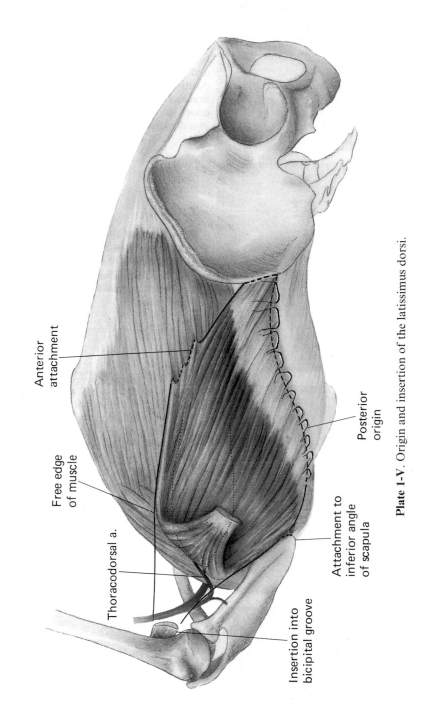

Anterior
attachment

Free edge
of muscle

Thoracodorsal a.

Insertion into
bicipital groove

Attachment to
inferior angle
of scapula

Posterior
origin

Plate 1-V. Origin and insertion of the latissimus dorsi.

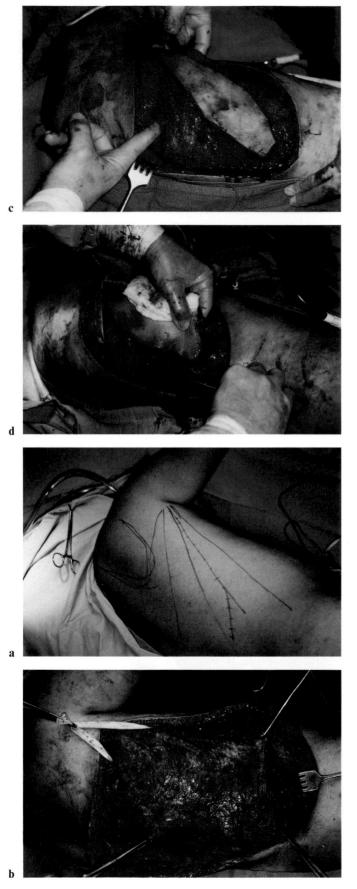

c. The anterior and posterior margins of the latissimus dorsi are dissected in the fashion described in Section 1.5.2.2.

d. The anterior margin is elevated and the muscle can be divided distally and posteriorly, depending on the amount required. It is important to ligate the vessels on the cut surface as the muscle is divided. If the entire muscle is taken, there will be less bleeding as the aponeurotic attachments are divided.

The remainder of the dissection is similar to that in Section 1.5.2.2.

1.5.2.4 Combined Latissimus Dorsi and Serratus Anterior Transplant (Harii et al. 1982) (Fig. 1-32)

a. The position used is similar to that described in Section 1.5.2.1. The incision is made approximately 4 cm posterior to the anterior margin of the latissimus dorsi.

b. The latissimus dorsi is dissected as described in Section 1.5.2.2, but the branch to the serratus anterior is *not* ligated.

c. The latissimus dorsi is elevated and the vessels are dissected back to the thoracodorsal vessels, which supply both muscles. The lowest digitations of the serratus anterior are then dissected as described in Section 1.5.2.1.

d. Further dissection proceeds into the axilla, dissecting the thoracodorsal vessels. Both muscles are then removed and are shown here, connected only by their vascular supply.

1.6 Tensor Fasciae Latae Musculocutaneous Transplant

(Cafee and Asokan 1981, Hill et al. 1978, Nahai et al. 1979)

1.6.1 Anatomy (Plate 1-VI)

The tensor fasciae latae muscle *arises* from the anterior part of the outer lip of the iliac crest and the outer surface of the anterior superior iliac spine. It is enclosed between the two layers of the fascia lata as it passes distally to *insert* into the iliotibial tract at the junction of the proximal and middle thirds of the thigh. Its *function* is that of a flexor, abductor, and medial rotator of the thigh, but its most important function is maintaining the extended knee in the erect position by keeping the iliotibial band taut.

The *vascular supply* to the muscle is from the lateral circumflex artery. This artery is a short vessel measuring a few centimeters in length and emanates from the profunda femoris artery. Thereafter, it gives off an ascending, a descending, and a transverse branch which becomes the pedicle to the tensor fasciae latae. This pedicle lies between the vastus lateralis and rectus femoris muscles approximately 8 cm distal to the iliac crest. It travels into the tensor fasciae latae muscle and divides into ascending, transverse, and descending branches which lie between the fascia and the muscle. It is the single dominant vessel to the muscle and is accompanied by two large venae comitantes. The artery rarely measures less than 1.5 mm in external diameter.

Perforating vessels pass from the muscle and fascia into the skin and allow a greater *cutaneous territory* to be supplied. This territory is distal to the muscle insertion and can reach approximately 8 cm from the lateral knee joint line (Mathes and Nahai 1979).

The lateral femoral cutaneous nerve is the *sensory supply* to the skin of the region (L2–L3). This nerve enters the area under the lateral end of the inguinal ligament. It can be superficial or deep to the sartorius. It lies deep to the fascia lata and becomes subcutaneous about 8 to 10 cm distal to the anterior superior iliac spine. There, it divides into anterior and posterior branches. A less important sensory supply proximally comes from the lateral cutaneous branch of T12, which enters the posterior aspect of the cutaneous flap.

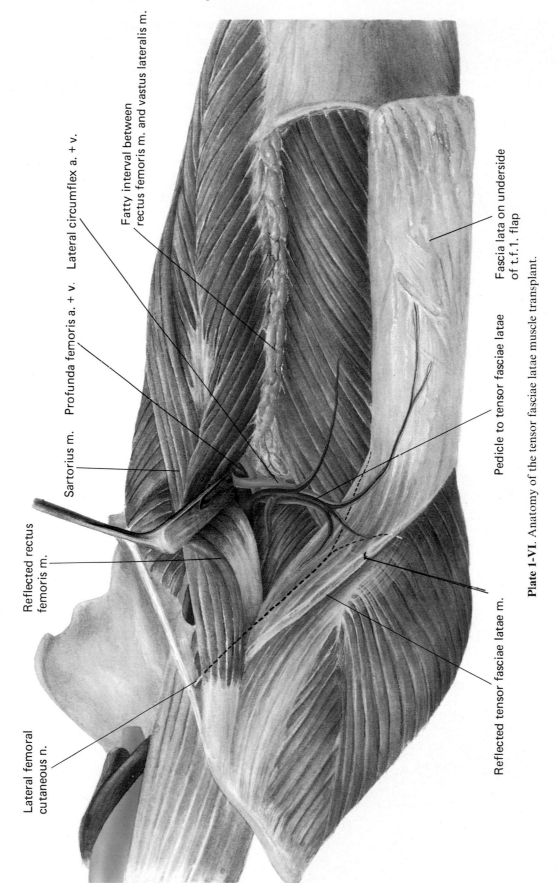

Fatty interval between rectus femoris m. and vastus lateralis m.

Lateral circumflex a. + v.

Profunda femoris a. + v.

Fascia lata on underside of t.f.1. flap

Sartorius m.

Pedicle to tensor fasciae latae

Reflected rectus femoris m.

Reflected tensor fasciae latae m.

Lateral femoral cutaneous n.

Plate 1-VI. Anatomy of the tensor fasciae latae muscle transplant.

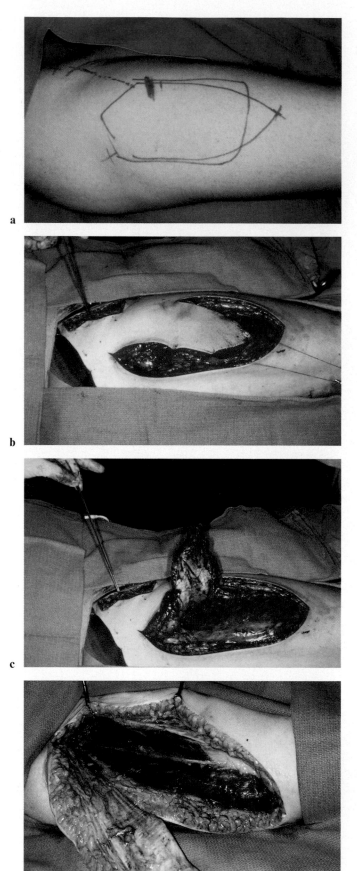

1.6.2 Surgical Technique
(Fig. 1-33; see also Fig. 1-21)

a. The skin incision which is outlined is centered proximally over the tensor fasciae latae, and distally along the anterolateral surface of the thigh. The anterior margin of this transplant runs from the anterior superior iliac spine to the lateral femoral condyle. The posterior margin parallels this line from the greater trochanter distally. If primary closure of the donor site is required, a narrower flap should be planned. Also, if the flap is not carried proximally to the iliac crest, donor site closure is easier. Distally, the flap can be extended to a point about 8 cm from the lateral knee joint line.

b. The lateral femoral cutaneous nerve is identified through a transverse incision that is made just distal to the lateral extent of the inguinal ligament. This nerve is then followed into the region of the proposed transplant. (Making an incision along the posterior and proximal margin of the flap, the lateral cutaneous branch of T12 can be dissected. This branch supplies the most proximal part of the flap and may sometimes be included.)

The skin incision is made laterally, medially, and distally down to the fascia lata. The skin is sutured to the fascia lata laterally, medially, and distally to prevent shearing of vessels between the skin superficially and the muscle and fascia.

c. The fascia lata is then incised, and the fascia and skin are elevated proximally as a unit.

d. As this flap is elevated, a fatty interval between the vastus lateralis and the rectus femoris becomes apparent. This fatty interval is shown in a cadaver dissection.

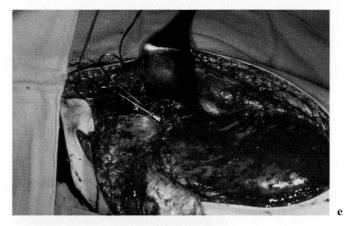

e. The pedicle is found within this interval 6–8 cm from the iliac crest. The vascular pedicle is dissected back to the origin from the lateral circumflex artery. The pedicle consists of two large venae comitantes and an artery.

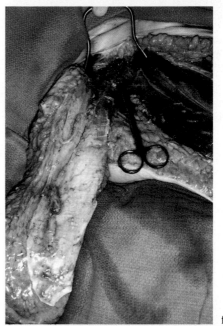

f. The pedicle is shown in this cadaver dissection.

g. The proximal dissection is then completed by either dividing the tensor fasciae latae proximally or separating the muscle from its origin at the outer border of the iliac crest. Care must be taken to find the plane that separates the gluteus minimus proximally and anteriorly.

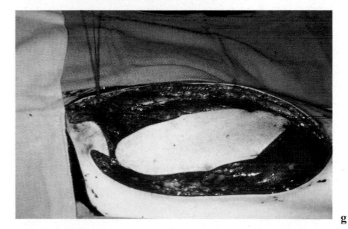

1.6.3 Donor Site Closure

a. If a flap 6–8 cm wide is taken, the donor site can usually be closed primarily. Closing the donor site too tightly may be dangerous because of the possibility of vascular compromise and consequent muscle necrosis.

b. If primary closure is not possible, a split-thickness skin graft is used on the muscle bed. Such skin grafting often has a poor cosmetic result because of a contour defect. If cosmetically unacceptable, the site can be treated secondarily with tissue expansion and subsequent graft removal.

1.7 Postoperative Care

Especially when split-thickness skin grafts have been used to cover a muscle transplant, it is important to apply *dressings* that contour the muscle well. Petroleum gauze followed by strips of cotton soaked in mineral oil will make such a dressing. Next, bulky gauze sponges are placed, followed by a plaster splint. A small opening is made in the skin graft to enable viewing of the muscle directly, and a window is left in all layers of the dressing for the same reason (Fig. 1-18).

No reliable surface *monitor* is currently available to monitor muscle tissue, but implanted temperature probes may be used to confirm the patency of the anastomoses (Fig. 8-2e). *Clinical observation* is usually adequate to assess whether the muscle is healthy and beefy red, or whether there is a vascular problem. Fortunately, it is unusual for a muscle transplant to develop vascular problems if vascularity has been adequate and

muscle color has been good during the first 12–18 hours after surgery.

Low-molecular-weight dextran (30 cc/hour for approximately 3 days) is used as an *anticoagulant*. Particular attention is devoted to ensuring that *hydration* is good and that body and ambient *temperature* are warm. Heparin should not be used, as it will often result in a hematoma at the donor site, probably because of the extensive raw surface area following this kind of procedure. The suction drain placed in the donor site should not be removed for 24 hours after the dextran has been discontinued – a precaution which is also aimed at preventing hematoma formation.

Continuous elevation for two weeks is imperative. This requisite is followed by a slow program of progressive dependency, starting with 10–15 minutes at a time. For 3 months an elastic bandage is worn whenever the extremity is dependent. If the transplant becomes congested or blue, the periods of dependency must be reduced.

1.8 Selected Bibliography

Bailey BN, Godfrey AM (1982) Latissimus dorsi muscle free flaps. Br J Plast Surg 35:47

Uses of the latissimus dorsi free flap in nine patients (in the lower extremity in seven cases, and one case each in the hand and head) are described. The benefits at the donor and recipient sites of using the muscle without overlying skin are discussed.

Byrd HS, Spicer TE, Cierney G III (1985) Management of open tibial fractures. Plast Reconstr Surg 76:719

A prospective, nonrandomized study of 73 type III and type IV open fractures treated with open-wound techniques or muscle flaps is reported. Early acute flap coverage provided the best results and had a lower complication rate than did open-wound techniques. Aggressive and repeated debridement is emphasized with the goal of flap coverage before wound colonization. Subacute wounds – those colonized and infected within 1 to 6 weeks of the injury – did relatively poorly with flap coverage, whereas chronic wounds with granulation fared better with this technique.

Cafee HH, Asokan R (1981) Tensor fascia lata myocutaneous free flaps. Plast Reconstr Surg 68:195

The advantages and disadvantages of this flap are described, based on the authors' experience with 12 transplants. The territory of the cutaneous flap, the problem of excessive bulk, and other technical aspects of the procedure are discussed.

Fisher J, Cooney WP III (1983) Designing the latissimus dorsi free flap for knee coverage. Ann Plast Surg 11:554

The technique of using the latissimus dorsi musculocutaneous free flap for knee coverage is described. The superficial femoral artery and vein are used as recipient vessels, and excess muscle is used to pack into the knee defect while cutaneous cover distally and over the knee is achieved.

Godina M (1986) Early microsurgical reconstruction of complex trauma of the extremities. Plast Reconstr Surg 78:285

A series of 532 patients who had undergone microsurgical reconstruction was divided into three groups: "early", "delayed", and "late" – designations which refer to the timing of the procedure. Flap failure, infection, bone healing time, and length of hospital stay were criteria used in evaluating the results. The infection rate among the free flaps that had been performed within 72 hours of injury (early) was only 1.5%. The flap failure rate in this group (0.75%) was also significantly lower than in the groups of patients who had undergone flap transfer at later stages (72 hours to 3 months later [delayed] –12%; 3 months to 12.6 years later [late] – 9.5%). Godina attributes this superior success rate to the absence of fibrosis, which makes procedure planning easier. Thorough wound debridement is emphasized.

Godina M, Bajec J, Baraga A (1986) Salvage of the mutilated upper extremity with temporary ectopic implantation of the undamaged part. Plast Reconstr Surg 78:295

Temporary "banking" of the hand in the axilla is described.

Gordon L, Buncke HJ, Alpert BS (1982) Free latissimus dorsi muscle flap with split-thickness skin graft cover: A report of 16 cases. Plast Reconstr Surg 70:173

This report describes using the latissimus dorsi muscle covered with a split-thickness skin graft instead of a musculocutaneous flap. Using split-thickness skin graft results in less bulk at the recipient site and superior donor site appearance.

Gordon L, Chiu E (1988) Treatment of infected nonunions and segmental defects of the tibia with staged microvascular muscle transplantation and bone grafting. J Bone Joint Surg 70-A:377

Most cases of chronic osteomyelitis combined with soft-tissue wounds can be controlled by appropriate bone and soft-tissue debridement, antibiotics, and microvascular muscle transplantation. The bone reconstruction that follows carries substantial risk of recurrent infection. In the humerus, femur, or where both bones have a segmental defect, vascularized bone transplantation should follow the muscle procedure after an infection-free interval. If the fibula is intact, however, a tibiofibular synostosis should be considered.

Gordon L, Rosen J, Alpert BS, et al (1984) Free microvascular transfer of second toe ray and serratus anterior muscle for management of thumb loss at the carpometacarpal joint level. J Hand Surg 9A(5):642

The second toe was used to reconstruct a thumb that had been previously amputated at the trapezium level. Absent thenar muscles were reconstructed with the serratus anterior.

Harii K, Ohmori K, Torii S (1976) Free gracilis muscle transplantation with microneurovascular anastomosis for the treatment of facial paralysis. A preliminary report. Plast Reconstr Surg 57:133

The anatomy and technique of gracilis transplantation are described.

Harii K, Yamada A, Ishihara K, et al (1982) A free transfer of both latissimus dorsi and serratus anterior flaps with thoracodorsal vessel anastomoses. Plast Reconstr Surg 70:620

The vascular anatomy of the two muscles as well as the surgical technique of flap elevation are described. This technique is useful in extremely large wounds where either the size of the latissimus dorsi is inadequate or dead space needs to be filled with muscle at the same time cover is provided. Donor site function is discussed.

Hill H, Nahai F, Vasconez L (1978) The tensor fascia lata myocutaneous free flap. Plast Reconstr Surg 61:517

Details of the anatomy and elevation of the flap are described. Six patients in whom this transplant was used are featured; three of the flaps contained a nerve, and four required debulking. Other advantages and disadvantages of this flap are discussed.

Manktelow RT, McKee NH (1979) Free muscle transplantation to provide active finger flexion. J Hand Surg 3:416

This article describes two patients who sustained traumatic loss of the long flexors to the digits. In both, flexor function was restored using free muscle transplantation – with the gracilis in one patient and the pectoralis major in the other. The *details* of each operative procedure are given and the functional results of the full range of flexion and grip strength are described. Also included is a discussion of some guidelines for performing the procedure.

Mathes SJ, Alpert BS, Chang N (1982) Use of the muscle flap in chronic osteomyelitis. Experimental and clinical correlation. Plast Reconstr Surg 69:815

This article reviews 11 patients with chronic osteomyelitis of the distal tibia and foot who were treated with debridement and gracilis muscle transplantation. An experimental model in the dog was used to compare musculocutaneous flaps with random-pattern cutaneous flaps. Possible reasons for the success of muscle flaps are given. The advantages of gracilis transplantation are discussed and operative technique is described.

Mathes SJ, Nahai F (1979) Clinical Atlas of Muscle and Musculocutaneous Flaps. St. Louis, C.V. Mosby

This outstanding volume presents the gamut of muscle flaps available for local or distant transfer.

Mathes SJ, Nahai F (1981) Classification of the vascular anatomy of muscles: Experimental and clinical correlation. Plast Reconstr Surg 67:177

This article is important reading for those involved in muscle transplantation. An anatomic study of the vascularity of different muscles is given with classification into five types of arterial supply. The importance of the vascular supply is correlated with clinical considerations in muscle transplantation.

Maxwell GP, Manson PN, Hoopes JE (1979) Experience with 13 latissimus dorsi myocutaneous free flaps. Plast Reconstr Surg 64:1

The vascular anatomy of the latissimus dorsi is described and the details of surgical technique are outlined. The possibility of "delay" of the flap and preliminary ligation of intercostal perforators are mentioned. Five cases are described in detail. The uses are listed and the donor site is discussed.

May JW Jr, Gallico GG III, Jupiter J, et al (1984) Free latissimus dorsi muscle flap with skin graft for treatment of traumatic chronic bony wounds. Plast Reconstr Surg 73:641

This use of the latissimus dorsi microvascular transplant is described. Indications and technique are outlined.

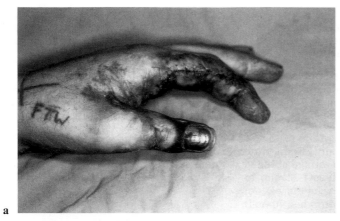

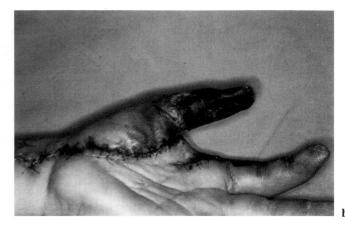

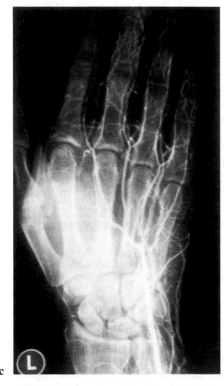

Fig. 2-1. a and **b.** A 19-year-old boy injected methylphenidate HCl into his radial artery at the midforearm level. Necrosis of the thumb and part of the radial aspect of the index finger resulted, along with inflammation on the dorsal aspect of the hand. Thin skin was needed to resurface the thumb and retain as much of its length as possible. It was also important to use a flap with good sensory innervation. Neither a radial forearm flap nor a rotation flap from the dorsum of the hand was possible in this patient because of the injury to the radial artery. A dorsalis pedis flap was used, as it best suited the patient's complex needs. **c.** Arteriography revealed an ulnar artery that supplied the ulnar three fingers and the ulnar aspect of the index finger. (It is important to recognize that the radial artery sometimes provides the only circulation to the thumb, index, and long fingers.) In light of this finding, the palmar arch was felt to be the safest recipient vessel. **d.** The necrotic tissue was removed, and the mummified portion of the thumb was amputated at the interphalangeal joint. The digital nerve was dissected to the base of the thumb where it had become necrotic. The superficial palmar arch was dissected as well as the median nerve, preserving the recurrent branch. The dorsalis pedis artery was sutured end-to-side into the superficial palmar arch, the vein was sutured end-to-end into the venae comitantes of the palmar arch, and the digital nerve was sutured to the superficial peroneal nerve. **e.** The flap is shown in place. A skin graft has been used on the radial aspect of the thumb. (Compared with skin grafting at the dorsalis pedis flap donor site, which can produce long-term healing problems, it is preferable to use a skin graft in the hand; this is especially true in this region of the thumb which is not directly involved in pinch or grip.) At 3 months, good sensation has been restored in the flap.

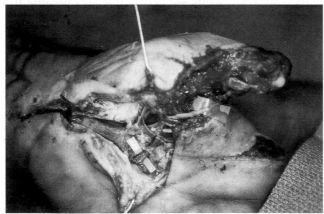

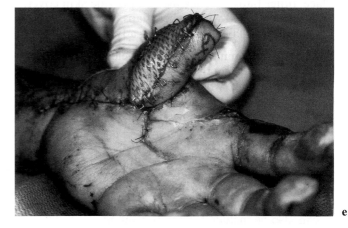

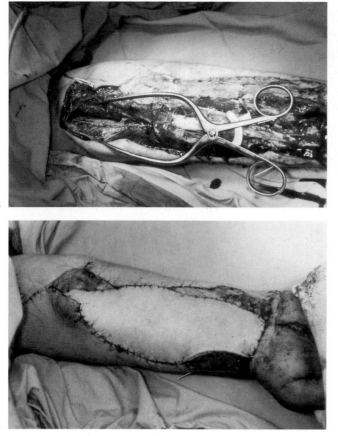
a

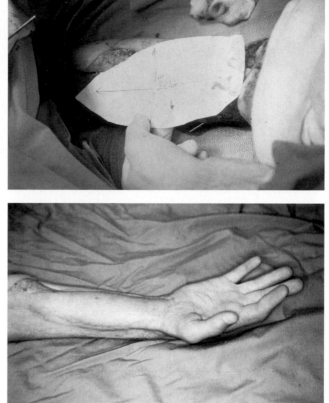
b

c

d

Fig. 2-2. a. Replantation was performed after an avulsive injury that involved amputation of the hand. Subsequently, a large cutaneous flap was needed to cover this extensive defect of the forearm which exposed the median nerve, radial artery, and many tendons of the flexor compartment. The radial vascular bundle was dissected proximally in order to provide the recipient vessels. **b.** A template of the wound was made so that a flap of appropriate dimensions could be harvested. **c.** Although the flap was shaped carefully to fit the defect, a small amount of skin graft was needed distally. **d.** The flap provided excellent cover and restored good function.

muscle coverage with a split-thickness skin graft tends to break down, and excessive scarring is often a problem. Musculocutaneous flaps can also be used in these areas (Fig. 1-26).

2.3 Choice of Transplant

A good microvascular cutaneous transplant must meet several criteria. For most defects, the skin should be thin (no excess subcutaneous fat) and large enough to cover the defect without excessive tension. The pedicle should be easy to dissect and have reliable anatomy, and its external diameter should be 1.5 mm or larger. The need for a long vascular pedicle will depend on the recipient site. In general, however, a pedicle at least 5 cm in length will allow the anastomosis to be performed more simply, away from the transplant, and with recipient vessels that are outside of the zone of injury. In addition, the donor site should be located in an inconspicuous area that can be closed primarily and not require skin grafting.

Skin flaps from almost every part of the body (the deltoid region; posterior, medial, and lateral arm; radial forearm; posterior and medial thigh; posterior and lateral calf; dorsum of the foot; instep; groin; and even the temporoparietal region) have been used to provide cutaneous soft-tissue cover. The two flaps that have achieved widespread acceptance because of the best overall combination of assets are the **lateral arm flap** (Figs. 2-3, 2-5, and 2-6) and the **scapular flap** (Figs. 2-2 and 2-4). When cutaneous soft-tissue cover is required, these two flaps can address any clinical contingency. The lateral arm flap provides some sensation and consists of thinner skin. The choice of cutaneous flap depends also on the *size of the defect*, as follows:

1. Defects measuring 2–3 cm × 6–8 cm – dorsalis pedis flap
2. Defects measuring up to 6–8 cm × 10–12 cm – lateral arm flap
3. Defects measuring 8–10 cm × 14–16 cm – scapular flap
4. Defects larger than 10 cm × 16 cm – latissimus dorsi musculocutaneous flap.

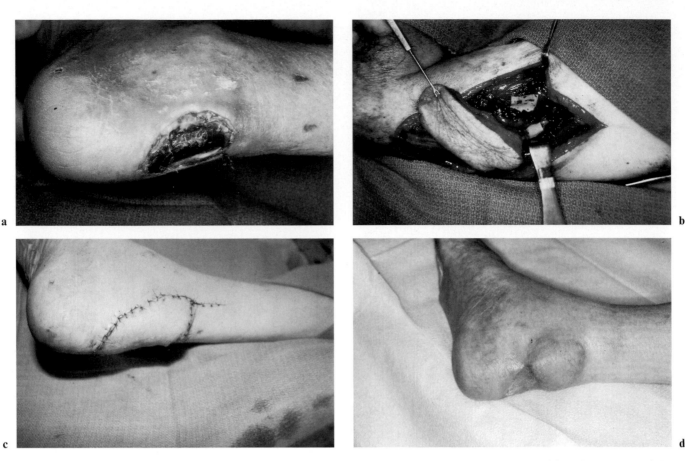

Fig. 2-3. a. An 80-year-old man with severe vascular disease developed this ulcer over his Achilles tendon. Loss of the Achilles tendon was imminent and the wound was not amenable to a local flap procedure. **b.** A lateral arm flap was harvested. The pedicle can be seen under the blue background. **c.** The vessels were anastomosed to the posterior tibial artery and vein. (Vessels in patients with diabetes and peripheral vascular disease must be sutured very carefully, passing the needle from the inside to the outside of the vessel so that the intima is not separated.) The flap of skin is thin and can be seen placed in the defect. **d.** The flap provided good cover 1 year later.

The lateral arm flap can be taken with an extension of the triceps fascia. This approach extends the area that can be covered with this flap, but the fascial extension requires split-thickness skin grafting. Some sensation in the flap is made possible by transplanting the lower lateral cutaneous nerve of the upper arm with it, but in my experience, the sensation restored is generally only fair. An insensate area over the lateral aspect of the elbow can be expected.

Katsaros and Schusterman (1984) have described the possible addition of bone or the use of the triceps fascia alone without overlying skin. The modification of taking fascia alone and using it for reconstruction in the lower extremity is appealing. Use of the humerus as part of an osteocutaneous transplant carries the risk of fracture at the donor site. These considerations must be carefully evaluated in relation to the many other options for bone transplantation.

Care should be taken not to close this wound too tightly. Katsaros and Schusterman (1984) have described one case in which the wound was extended distal to the elbow and closed tightly. Postoperatively, the patient was found to have radial nerve compression which resolved once the sutures were released.

The scapular and lateral arm flaps are compared in Table 2-1.

Table 2-1. A comparison of the lateral arm and scapular flaps.

	Lateral arm flap	Scapular flap
Size	6–8 × 10–12 cm	8–10 × 14–16 cm
Vascular anatomy	Dependable	Dependable
Skin characteristics	Thin	Slightly thicker
Subcutaneous tissue	Little	Moderate (depends on body fat)
Pedicle length	6 cm	6 cm (with difficulty, can be extended to 10 cm)
Patient position	Supine	Prone or lateral
Donor site result	Linear scar; slight contour defect	Linear scar; tends to spread

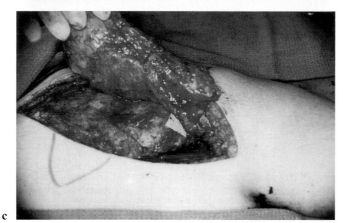

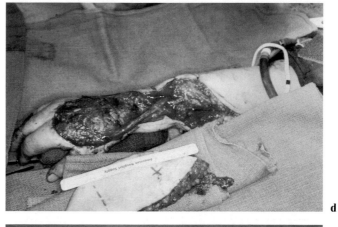

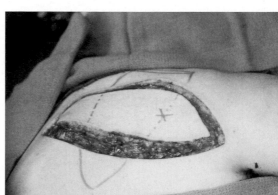

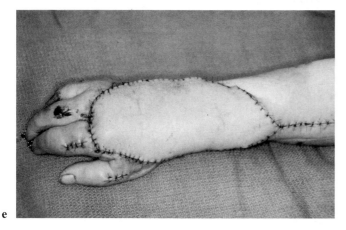

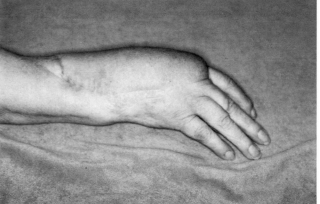

Fig. 2-4. a. A car rolled over onto this patient's hand and wrist, resulting in severe bone and soft-tissue loss at the wrist level. Wrist fusion was needed in addition to tendon reconstruction, and adequate soft-tissue cover was lacking. The patient is shown approximately 1 year after the accident. A flap was needed which would be wider than the lateral arm flap and contain more subcutaneous tissue so that it would fill the defect. It was felt that skin with subcutaneous tissue would allow for subsequent tendon gliding better than would muscle or fascial cover. For these reasons, the scapular flap was chosen. **b.** The scapula was outlined and the flap incised. The Doppler signal was marked. **c.** The flap was elevated; the blue background is beneath where the pedicle curves around the lateral border of the scapula through the triangular space. **d.** The defect was prepared and the proximal radial artery dissected as the recipient vessel. The flap measured 15 cm × 9 cm and had a 5-cm vascular pedicle. **e.** The flap was sutured into place, providing good cover. **f.** Improved contour was achieved with adequate cover for subsequent tendon reconstruction and wrist fusion.

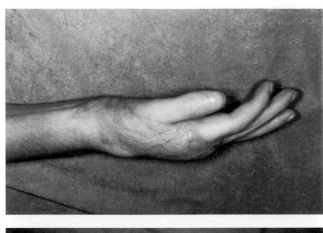

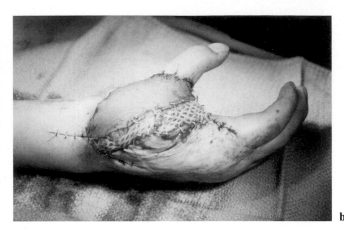

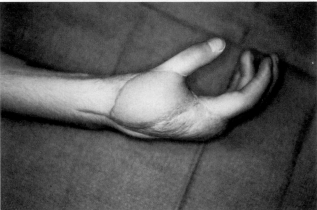

Fig. 2-5. a. This fixed adduction deformity, which was the
result of a severe crush injury to the dorsum and palm of
the hand, obstructed thumb function. This 12-year-old girl
was adamantly opposed to any procedure that would involve
scarring or skin grafting in the forearm or abdomen. The
lateral arm flap was an attractive alternative because of the
appearance of the donor site and its ability to provide thin
pliable skin. b. The flap was placed in the defect after the
web space was released. c. The final result.

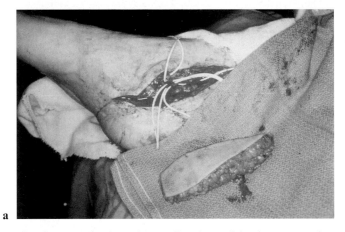

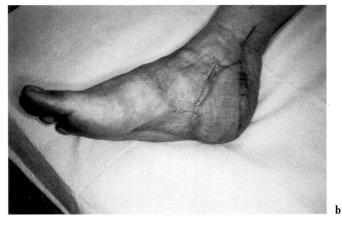

Fig. 2-6. a. The lateral arm flap is useful where sensation
is important, such as on the sole of the foot. In this patient,
a split-thickness skin graft had been performed to cover the
entire heel after an injury there. Subsequently, intermittent
breakdown occurred in the region. b. A lateral arm flap was
used to provide sensation and good full-thickness cover.

Fig. 2-7. a. A 24-year-old laborer suffered a crushing amputation of all his fingers. Good soft-tissue cover with sensate skin was needed. A "retrograde" radial forearm flap measuring 12 cm × 10 cm was indicated (see also Fig. 2-13). **b.** Sensation was restored (*shaded areas*) by suturing the lateral cutaneous nerve of the forearm to the common digital nerves of the index and long fingers. **c.** Good grasp was restored. (Courtesy of Hill Hastings II.)

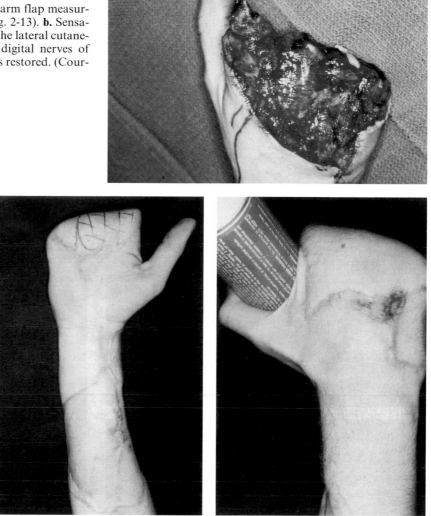

The **dorsalis pedis flap** (McCraw and Furlow 1975, Zuker and Manktelow 1985) (Fig. 2-1) provides good thin skin but is quite small. Its main advantage is that it includes a nerve and can provide sensory return. Skin grafting is required if a flap wider than 3 cm is taken, in which case the donor site can present problems with discomfort and breakdown. If a flap wider than 3 cm is needed, donor site problems make this flap undesirable compared with other skin flaps that allow primary donor site closure in less critical areas (Fig. 2-8).

The utility of this flap is greatest when it accompanies the metatarsophalangeal joint or the metatarsal and tendon as a composite tissue transplant (Fig. 4-19). In this circumstance, a narrow flap is usually sufficient and primary closure of the donor site is possible. The dorsalis pedis flap may be tailored to specific problems in the hand (Fig. 2-1) and may include skin from the dorsum of the foot with extensions distally on one or both sides of the first web space (Fig. 2-9); this may be useful in some hand defects (Doi and Hattorii 1980).

This flap is particularly indicated where sensation is important.

In 3–7% of patients, the dorsalis pedis artery emanates from the peroneal artery (Fig. 1-23; Plate 4-V). Also, the first dorsal metatarsal artery is variable (Plate 4-IV). Arteriography and Doppler studies should confirm the anatomy of the dorsalis pedis and first dorsal metatarsal arteries (Man and Acland 1980, see comments by Banis in Zuker and Manktelow 1985).

The **radial forearm flap** (Mühlbauer et al. 1982, Song et al. 1982) (Fig. 2-7) is based on the radial artery, and provides thin pliable skin. This flap is relatively large and the anatomy of the vessels is constant, making dissection easy. However, the donor site requires skin grafting and may be unsightly because of its location in an exposed region. By including the lateral and/or the medial cutaneous nerve of the forearm, a flap with sensation can be achieved. In rare circumstances, a part of the radius, the brachioradialis, or flexor carpi radialis can also be included. Removal of a corticocancellous

Mühlbauer W, Herndl E, Stock W (1982) The forearm flap. Plast Reconstr Surg 70:336

The history, surgical technique, and clinical uses of the radial forearm flap are described. These authors prefer immediate reconstruction of the radial artery with a reversed vein graft.

Nassif TM, Vidal L, Bovet JL, et al (1982) The parascapular flap. A new cutaneous microsurgical free flap. Plast Reconstr Surg 69:591

The axis of this flap, which is based on the descending branch of the circumflex scapular artery, follows the lateral border of the scapula. This flap demonstrates the versatility of the tissue supplied by the subscapular artery, and the article emphasizes combinations of the scapular flap, parascapular flap, and latissimus dorsi transplant. The anatomy and surgical technique are described in detail.

Russell RC, Guy RJ, Zook EG, et al (1985) Extremity reconstruction using the free deltoid flap. Plast Reconstr Surg 76:586

The detailed anatomy and technique of raising this flap are given. The area of sensation averages 15 cm × 10 cm. Results in ten clinical cases where the flap measured 4 cm × 6 cm to 33 cm × 13 cm are described. The authors emphasize that inclusion of a sensory nerve is an advantage, and they used this flap on the palm and dorsum of the hand as well as in the heel.

Song R, Gao Y, Song Y, et al (1982) The forearm flap. Clin Plast Surg 9:21

This paper discusses the anatomic basis of the forearm flap, and provides the details of dissection.

Upton J, Rogers C, Durham-Smith G, et al (1986) Clinical applications of free temporoparietal flaps in hand reconstruction. J Hand Surg 11A:475

Vascularized temporoparietal fascia was used for defects in the hand or fingers that measured up to 14 cm × 12 cm. Technique and clinical applications are discussed. The variations in anatomy of the superficial temporal artery are important.

Urbaniak J, Koman LA, Goldner RD, et al (1982) The vascularized cutaneous scapular flap. Plast Reconstr Surg 69:772

The anatomy and surgical technique are explained in detail, and five clinical cases involving the lower extremities are described.

Zuker RM, Manktelow RT (1985) The dorsalis pedis free flap. Technique of elevation, foot closure, and flap applications. Plast Reconstr Surg 77:93

The dorsalis pedis flap is described for reconstruction of the heel and the hand where innervation is important. Anatomy and technique are outlined clearly and in detail. In this series of 45 patients, the vascular anatomy was found to be reliable. The primary disadvantage of this procedure lies in the donor site if too broad a flap is taken for primary foot closure. The details of skin grafting and care of the donor site are included. (Further analysis of this flap is found in the accompanying discussion of the article by Dr. Joseph C. Banis, who addresses the anatomic variability of the dorsalis pedis artery.)

3.1 Overview

The many bone grafting methods which surgeons have used over the years have utilized a graft that serves primarily as a matrix with relatively few surviving osseous cells. Ostrup and Fredrickson (1974) were the first to scientifically investigate the fate of bone cells in grafts when circulation to the grafted bone could be maintained. Later, others confirmed experimentally that, under such conditions, osteocytes will survive, obviating the slow process of creeping substitution whereby dead bone is replaced by living bone (Berggren et al. 1982). The applicability of this experimental work to clinical cases continues to be a subject of spirited investigation.

This chapter deals with situations where nonvascularized bone grafts are likely to fail because of slow or absent bone healing. When faced with such problems, vascularized bone grafting provides an attractive alternative. To a great extent, bone healing relies on the ingrowth of vascularity from the surrounding bed. A nonvascularized graft may fail when used in a poorly vascularized bone graft bed or in abnormal bone, which is why vascularized bone grafts are advocated for irradiated or infected areas and areas with extensive fibrosis. In these situations, better healing is likely with the use of bone that has an independent vascular supply.

3.2 Indications

3.2.1 Congenital Problems – Inherent Bone
Pathology (Gordon et al. 1986, Pho et al. 1985, Weiland et al. 1987)

Congenital pseudarthrosis of the tibia is a poorly understood problem in which healing of the tibia is difficult to secure and maintain. There is strong clinical evidence that *healing can be achieved earlier* (usually within 3 months of transplantation) and *hypertrophy attained more rapidly* with vascularized bone transplantation than with other techniques (Fig. 3-1); in several centers, 5- to 10-year results are now available, confirming the usefulness of this technique (Weiland et al. 1987). The operation takes 4–5 hours and is straightforward and reliable. The sole disadvantage is that the *donor leg* is left with a single bone. (A synostosis between the tibia and what remains of the distal fibula will prevent ankle valgus in the donor leg.) Patients with this condition must be followed to skeletal maturity to ensure that pseudarthrosis does not recur.

3.2.2 Traumatic Bone Defects
(Taylor 1983, Weiland et al. 1979, Wood 1986)

In treating *extensive traumatic bone defects*, healing and hypertrophy can often be obtained earlier with vascularized bone transplantation than with nonvascularized grafting. However, other treatment options such as allograft replacement or conventional (nonvascularized) bone grafting must also be considered.

The disadvantages of bone allografts are their high rate of infection, fatigue fracture, and nonunion (Mankin et al. 1983). This is especially true where there has been prior infection, fibrosis, or poor blood supply – conditions under which healing is also likely to be slow. Allografts have been used extensively after tumor resection. The remaining tissues are generally of better quality in these cases than they are following trauma. Fatigue fractures of allografts generally heal poorly, whereas similar fractures of vascularized bone tend to heal rapidly.

Conventional bone grafts from the iliac crest and other, more recently developed bone substitutes can sometimes achieve osseous integrity for *short defects*. The difficulty arises in establishing a cut-off length above which vascularized bone transplantation is preferable, but below which conventional bone grafting techniques will suffice. Clearly, no absolute cut-off ex-

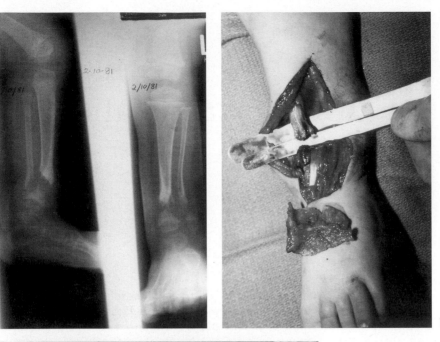

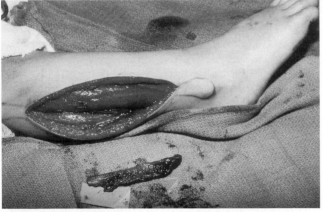

Fig. 3-1. a. A 26-month-old girl had been diagnosed with congenital pseudarthrosis of the tibia (Boyd, type 2) at 2 weeks of age. The pseudarthrosis was near the ankle joint, and the unfavorable radiographic appearance is shown. b. It is important to debride the abnormal bone and soft tissue in the region of the pseudarthrosis. The tibia was resected back to healthy, bleeding bone where a medullary cavity was present. The anterior tibial vessels were dissected (they are easy to expose on the lateral aspect of the tibia). c. The donor fibula was dissected. The vascular pedicle is seen under the blue background.

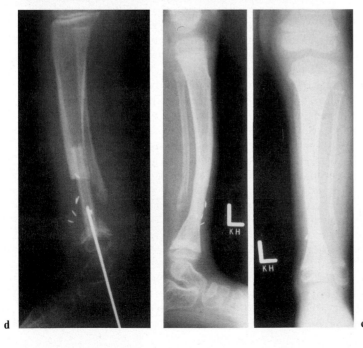

Fig. 3-1. d. The vascularized fibula transplant was placed in the medullary canal of the tibia proximally. Because fixation to the very soft distal tibial fragment was difficult, an intramedullary Kirschner wire was used to hold the transplant in place. e. Solid healing and good hypertrophy of the transplant were achieved by 5 months. In an incident 2 years after the transplant, the patient discarded her brace and jumped from a 6-foot height, fracturing her tibia; the fracture healed uneventfully in an interval similar to that expected for a normal bone. At follow-up 5 years later, solid healing had been maintained.

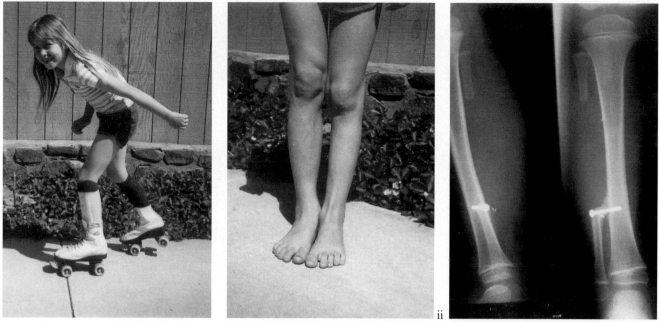

fi
ii
g

Fig. 3-1. f. i and ii. At the time of this photograph, the patient was 7 years old and fully active. Her left knee was slightly more distal than her right. A brace will be worn until she reaches skeletal maturity. **g.** In the donor leg, a tibiofibular synostosis was done between the remaining fibula and the tibia. (At least the distal fourth of the fibula should be retained.) (I thank Dr. Harry Jergesen for his expert orthopaedic care of this patient.)

ists, and this length varies, depending on the philosophy, expertise, and training of the surgeon. The condition of the recipient bed and the demands on the recipient bone must be evaluated. These factors require that an individualized decision be made for each patient.

It is important that each surgeon establish clear indications for vascularized bone transplantation. The following discussion outlines my protocol.

3.2.2.1 Extensive Bone Defect: No Intact Bone

For defects of the humerus (Fig. 3-2), femur (Fig. 3-3), or both bones of the forearm or leg (Fig. 3-4) that are longer than approximately 5 cm, vascularized fibula transplantation may be indicated, depending on the graft bed (Jupiter et al. 1987). Allografts should be considered if there has not been previous infection, but most posttraumatic defects have a great deal of fibrosis and the condition of the soft tissue is poor. Vascularized fibula transplantation has the advantage of early healing and rapid hypertrophy. The worse the bone graft bed, the more attractive vascularized bone transplantation becomes.

A similar philosophy applies to very long tibial defects in which there has been previous infection, even if the fibula is intact, because the additional support of the transplanted fibula may be important. An infection-free interval of 3–6 months is required following debridement if bone grafting is to be done relatively safely (Fig. 3-5).

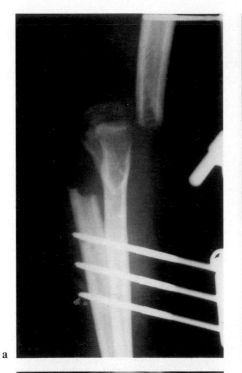

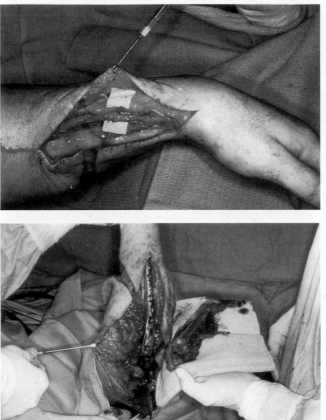

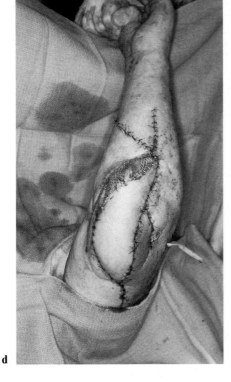

Fig. 3-2. a. A 36-year-old man lost his distal humerus, elbow joint, and proximal radius in a car accident. There was severe muscle damage, *soft-tissue cover* posteriorly was inadequate for extensive bone grafting, and the surrounding area was fibrotic. In addition to the *cortical bone defect*, there was poor cancellous bone. An elbow fusion was planned. Both corticocancellous bone and soft-tissue cover were needed. After considering these deficiencies and the fact that vascularized bone can enable the earliest healing possible, an iliac crest osteocutaneous transplant made the most attractive treatment option. **b.** The radial artery and venae comitantes were dissected distally, divided near the wrist, and swung across the volar surface of the forearm to be used as the recipient vessels; this was preferable to using the brachial artery, the proximal radial artery, or the ulnar artery. Not only would these options have required extensive vein grafting, but use of the brachial or ulnar artery involves greater risk to the hand circulation. **c.** The plate was placed to provide stability, but a bone defect remained between the ulna and humerus, and the soft-tissue defect with the exposed plate was evident. This photograph shows the flap, which is based on the deep circumflex iliac vessel and contains a portion of the iliac crest and overlying groin skin. **d.** Two lagged cortical screws were used to fix both ends of the bone transplant, and the cutaneous flap was sutured into place.

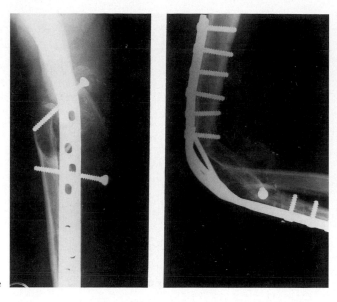

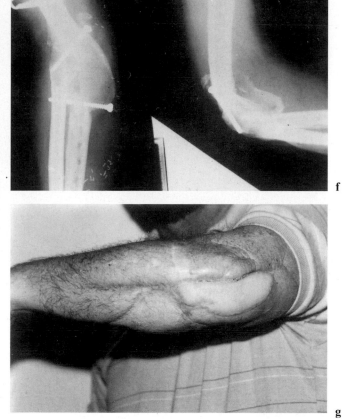

Fig. 3-2e. Postoperative radiographs. **f.** Final result. Radiographs show the position of the bone graft, which was well healed by 3 months and allowed plate removal at 7 months. **g.** The cutaneous portion of the transplant provides good cover.

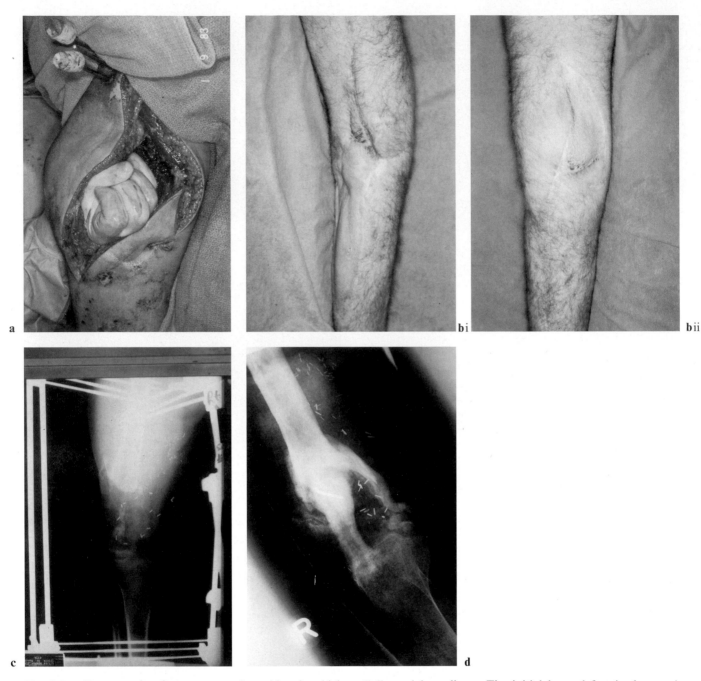

Fig. 3-3. a. Four months after a motorcycle accident in which this patient lost a substantial amount of his distal femur, he developed a gram-negative infection. The wound was thoroughly debrided, leaving an extensive through-and-through soft-tissue defect in the distal thigh and knee region. **b.** i and ii. A latissimus dorsi muscle transplant was used to fill the through-and-through soft-tissue defect and provide cover medially and laterally. **c.** The initial bone defect is shown. A fibula transplant was chosen over an allograft because of the extensive fibrosis and previous infection. **d.** Eighteen months later, marked hypertrophy of the bone graft with solid healing at both ends was demonstrated on radiography; this degree of healing allowed the patient to be fully weight bearing in a brace.

Fig. 3-4. a. A segmental defect of the tibia and fibula resulting from a gunshot wound was combined with a severe soft-tissue wound. A muscle transplant was used to provide soft-tissue cover. **b.** The bone defect is shown here. A single vessel, the posterior tibial, was present in this leg, necessitating an end-to-side anastomosis. **c.** A vascularized fibula transplant was placed in the intramedullary position proximally and distally in the tibia. **d** and **e.** Fourteen months later, solid healing and hypertrophy of the vascularized fibula transplant allowed the patient to be fully weight bearing.

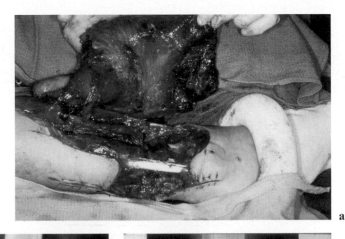

a

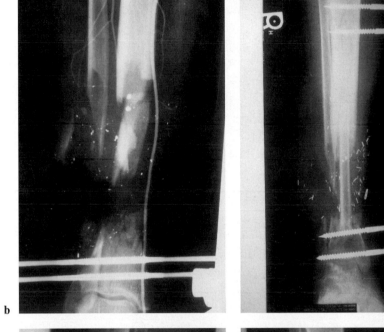

b

c

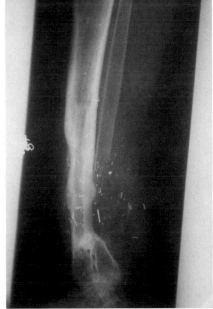

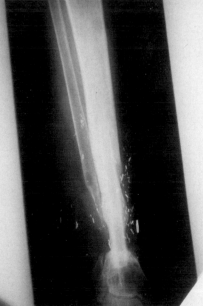

d

e

76

3. Vascularized Bone Transplantation

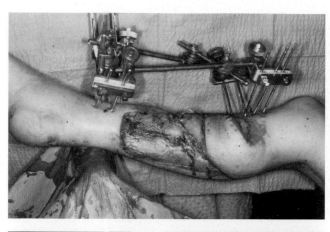

a

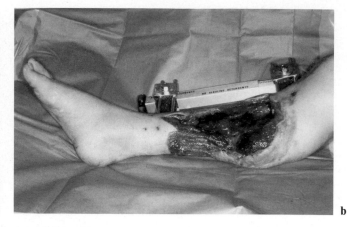

b

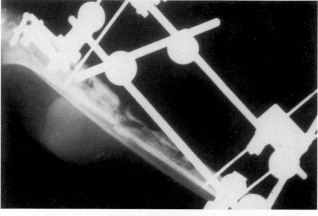

c

Fig. 3-5. a. This 32-year-old patient was referred after failure of a gastrocnemius-soleus pedicle flap. This flap was meant to cover an anterior tibial wound that resulted from a motorcycle accident. There was a gram-negative infection involving both bone and soft tissue. b. The pedicle flap was replaced in its original position and the area was meticulously debrided. The external fixator was also replaced to allow easier access to the posterior tibial vessels. (After osteomyelitis, it is wise to follow debridement with muscle transplantation and achieve a closed wound that shows no evidence of infection for several months before proceeding with bone transplantation or grafting.) c. The severely infected bone of the midtibia was not salvageable because it was intensely purulent.

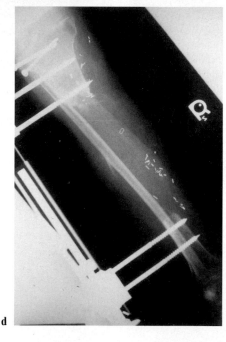

d

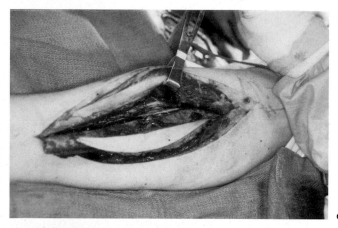

e

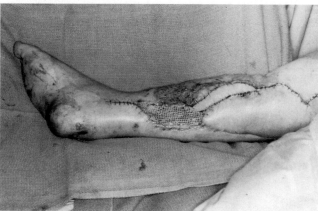

f

Fig. 3-5. d. Following debridement of the grossly infected bone, a large segmental tibial defect remained. e. The fibula transplant was harvested and it included an island of skin. f. The island of skin was used to confirm vascularity in the transplant.

Fig. 3-5. g. The vascularized fibula
transplant was placed in the defect.
After 14 months, the transplant had hypertrophied and the patient was initiated
on partial weight bearing in a cast brace.
At 17 months, he was fully weight bearing. h. Excellent soft-tissue cover and so-
lidly healed bone were ultimately
achieved.

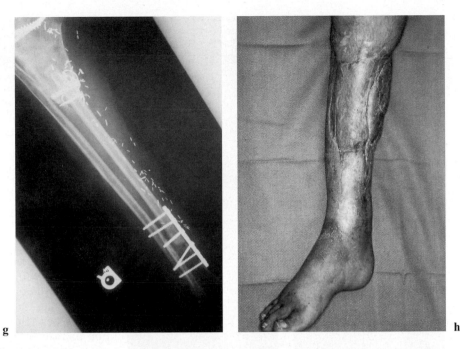

g

h

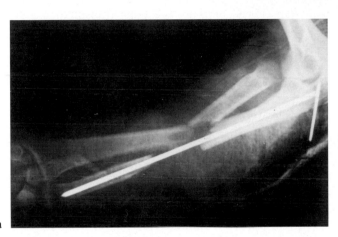

a

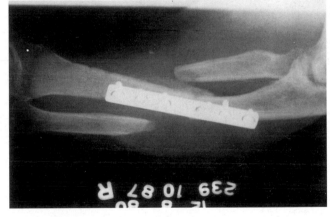

b

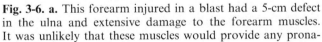

Fig. 3-6. a. This forearm injured in a blast had a 5-cm defect
in the ulna and extensive damage to the forearm muscles.
It was unlikely that these muscles would provide any pronation or supination. b. A one-bone forearm was the best solution in this patient.

3.2.2.2 Extensive Bone Defect: One Intact Bone

A *tibial defect with an intact fibula* holds the possibility
of regaining osseous integrity through the fibula. The
techniques of proximal and distal tibiofibular synostosis (Fig. 1-13c) and vascular pedicle grafting using the
ipsilateral fibula should be considered (Chacha et al.
1981, Maurer and Dillin 1987). These options may be
preferable to vascularized fibula transplantation,
especially if the site has been previously infected; in
my experience, there is a high incidence of postoperative infection when vascularized bone grafting is done
in such a previously infected area. If there has been
previous osteomyelitis and the fibula is intact, then vascularized fibula transplantation is less desirable. In the
absence of previous infection, however, vascularized

fibula transplantation supplemented with cancellous
bone grafting will usually effect rapid bone healing.
In such situations, vascularized bone grafting, allograft-
ing, or tibiofibular synostosis may be appropriate, depending on the bone graft bed (Sec. 3.2.2.1).

In the *forearm*, the fibula can successfully replace
the radius or ulna with the advantage of restoring
pronation and supination. If passive pronation and
supination or the muscles that produce these move-
ments are absent, vascularized fibula transplantation
is contraindicated and a one-bone forearm is preferable (Castle 1974) (Fig. 3-6). If the defect is in
the distal radius, proximal ulna, or both bones, a
one-bone forearm is not possible and vascularized
bone transplantation may then be indicated (Dell et al.
1984).

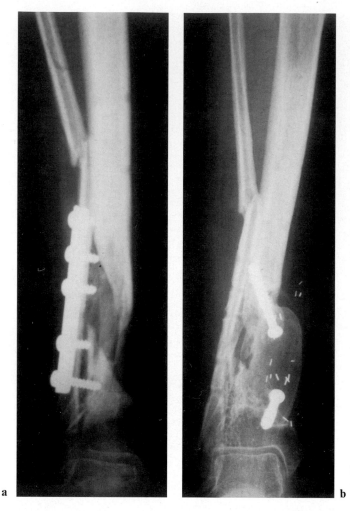

a

b

Fig. 3-7. a. A 40-year-old woman sustained severe injuries to her distal tibia in an automobile accident. Some stability was present, but there was severe soft-tissue injury, a bone gap with deformity of the fibula, and no evidence of healing a year after the injury despite bone grafting. Because there was some stability and the primary objective was to achieve bone healing, transplantation of vascularized iliac crest was preferred to fibula because of its higher cancellous bone content. A cutaneous flap was included to remedy the poor soft-tissue cover anteriorly. b. Two years later, solid healing of the graft enabled the patient to be fully weight bearing without aids.

⊲————————————————————————————————

3.2.2.3 Short Bone Defects With or Without Soft-Tissue Cover

For bone defects shorter than 4–5 cm, nonvascularized bone grafting techniques should usually be attempted first, with vascularized bone grafting being reserved for failures. Sometimes, bone healing does not occur despite the fact that the defect is relatively small. Nonunion may be the result of poor vascularity, and the addition of vascularized cancellous bone (vascularized iliac crest) may solve this problem (Fig. 3-7). A cutaneous skin flap can accompany the bone transplant if soft-tissue cover is poor (Fig. 3-8).

3.2.3 Defects Following Tumor Removal
(Moore et al. 1983)

Following bone resection for benign or malignant tumors, the remaining bed is generally of reasonably good quality, and ingrowth of vasculature from surrounding tissues and healing can be expected. In such cases, allografts are usually successful. Following irradiation, however, vascularized bone may be a better option because of the poor vascularity of the soft tissues. After irradiation or with extensive defects, vascularized fibula transplantation may be appropriate. An allograft may

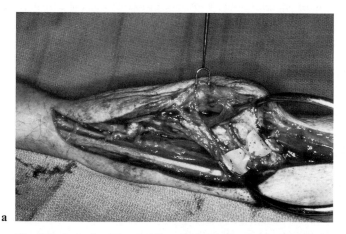

a

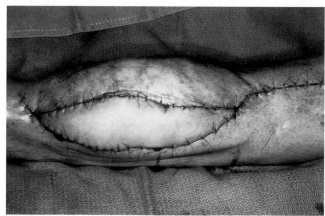

b

Fig. 3-8. (see also Fig. 3–12) a. This patient had a persistent tibial nonunion despite multiple bone grafting attempts. A latissimus dorsi muscle flap had been used to provide soft-tissue cover. The recipient vessels are shown and are the same ones that were used for the previous latissimus dorsi trans- plant. (After approximately 6 months, these vessels can be reused with little danger to the transplant – by then, the transplant can be expected to have established a second blood supply from the tissue bed.) b. The wound was covered and the vascularized bone used to bridge the nonunion site.

be combined with a vascularized bone graft from either the fibula or iliac crest. Currently, it is not clear whether the addition of vascularized bone lowers the nonunion rate or the fatigue failure rate after allograft procedures.

3.2.4 Spine Defects

Vascularized fibula transplantation for vertebral stability is promising. The strength of the fibula makes it attractive for this use. Its size allows easy fitting into the vertebra, and the intercostal or lumbar vessel can be used for vascular supply. Still, the long-term results of this application are yet to be seen (Fig. 3-9).

3.2.5 Avascular Necrosis of the Hip

Long-term results of vascularized fibula transplantation for avascular necrosis of the hip have not yet been published. Until such information is forthcoming, this application must be considered experimental.

3.2.6 Acetabular and Proximal Femur Reconstruction

Dissection of the iliac crest based on the deep circumflex iliac artery as an "island graft" will allow rotation of this vascularized bone, which can then be used to reconstruct the proximal femur or acetabulum (Leung and Chow 1984).

3.3 Choice of Transplant

Two vascularized bone transplants are used for extremity reconstruction: the fibula and the iliac crest (Chen and Yan 1983). Their important characteristics are compared in Table 3-1. The fibula is strong, straight, and long, and is therefore ideal for reconstructing major long bones. The donor site is generally benign. In skeletally immature individuals, a distal tibiofibular synostosis must be performed to prevent ankle valgus deformity. The iliac crest is curved, but has a large cancellous component, which is an advantage in promoting early osseous healing.

With these features in mind, the choice of transplant may be considered as follows.

Table 3-1. Comparison of the fibula and iliac crest transplants.

	Fibula transplant	Iliac crest transplant
Donor Site (Fig. 3-10)	Appearance excellent; tibiofibular synostosis required distally	Appearance good; hernia potential
Ease of dissection	Easy (1 hour)	Moderate to difficult (3 hours)
Bone length	5–25 cm (straight)	5–15 cm (surface curved if more than 8 cm is taken)
Pedicle	3–5 cm long with an external diameter of 1.5-3 mm	5–7 cm long with an external diameter of 1.5-3 mm
Bone type	Strong cortex; poorly cancellous	Weak cortex; primarily cancellous
Skin component	Small island of skin can accompany bone (frequently used as a vascular marker; utility for skin cover less well established [Yoshimura et al. 1983])	Large island of skin can accompany bone

Fibula

Used for most vascularized bone reconstruction in the extremities (Figs. 3-3 and 3-4)

For long bone replacement where bone strength is important and structural integrity needs to be restored

Iliac Crest

Used where some stability is present but osseous healing is needed (e.g., tibial nonunions that have repeatedly failed to heal by other methods) (Fig. 3-7)

Used where a curved surface is needed, e.g., for an elbow fusion (Fig. 3-2) – the iliac crest can be curved by a controlled "greenstick" fracture of the outer table, allowing bending of the bone to the appropriate shape

Used for osteocutaneous transplantation where both bone and soft-tissue cover are needed (Gordon et al. 1985, Taylor et al. 1979) (Fig. 3-2)

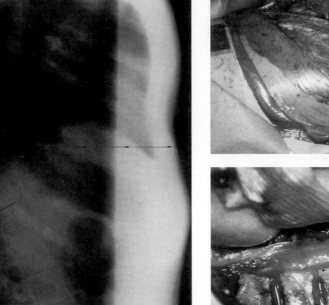

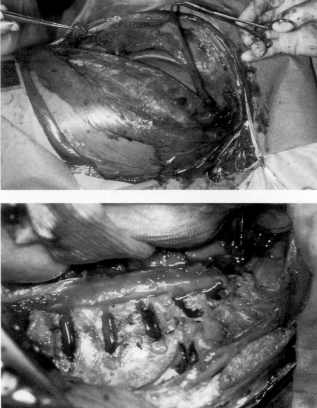

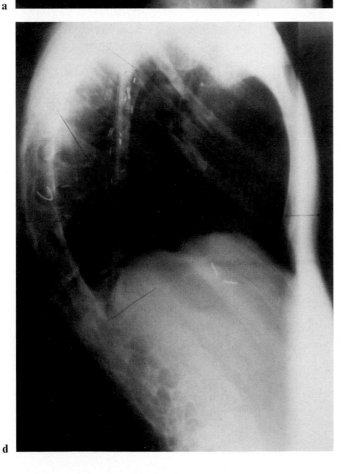

Fig. 3-9. (see also Fig. 3-11) **a.** This 13-year-old boy developed severe, progressive kyphosis following the resection of an astrocytoma from the thoracic spine. Following a laminectomy he developed instability with increasing kyphoscoliosis. The kyphosis measured 70°. As a first stage, a posterior fusion in situ with conventional iliac crest bone graft was performed. Bone grafting anteriorly was needed to provide strong support and achieve early healing in order to arrest the progress of the kyphosis. A vascularized fibula transplant was planned. **b.** The second stage was performed four weeks later. The thorax was entered through removal of T7, and the intercostal artery was dissected from this interspace for use as the recipient artery (*held up by clamp*). The hemiazygos vein was used as the recipient vein. **c.** The fibula transplant is seen in place, spanning the interval from T4 to T12. Twenty degrees of correction was obtained at the time of insertion of the fibula graft. **d.** Nine months later, the patient was asymptomatic but continued to wear a brace part time. The fibula graft healed at both ends, had hypertrophied, and can be seen here spanning the region of kyphosis, which has remained stable. (The spinal surgery was performed by John M. Gray, M.D.)

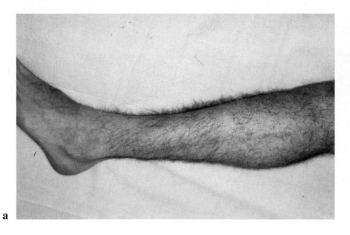

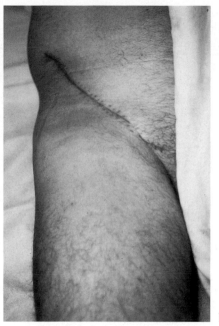

Fig. 3-10. a. The donor site following fibula transplantation is usually inconspicuous, and leg function is normal. **b.** The donor site following osteocutaneous groin transplantation is shown. Hernia formation is a potential complication (Sec. 3.5.2h). There are no functional problems in the extremity, but an area of numbness in the anterior thigh usually exists.

Table 3-2. Vascularized bone transplantation for traumatic bone defects of the lower extremity – indications.

Size of bone defect (cm)	Quality of graft bed	Graft indication
<4–5	favorable	nonvascularized bone
	unfavorable*	vascularized bone (iliac crest)
>4–5 (one intact bone)	favorable	allograft, vascularized fibula, or both
	unfavorable no prior infection	vascularized fibula
	prior infection	proximal and distal tibiofibular synostosis
>4–5 (no intact bone)	favorable	allograft, vascularized fibula, or both
	unfavorable	vascularized bone

* is fibrotic, irradiated, or has poor soft-tissue cover

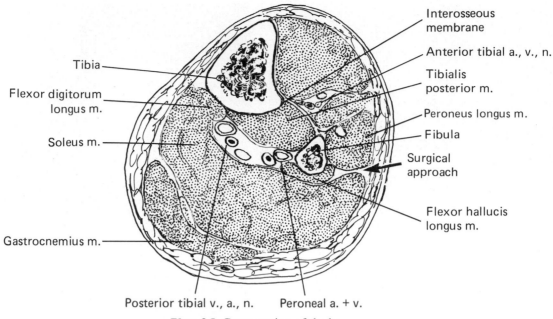

Plate 3-I. Cross section of the leg.

3.4 Vascularized Fibula Transplantation
(Chen and Yan 1983, Gilbert 1981, Taylor 1983, Taylor et al. 1975, Weiland et al. 1983, Wood 1986)

3.4.1 Anatomy (Plates 3-I and 3-II)

The *fibula* is a long, relatively straight and slender bone. It consists of an expanded head proximally, a body, and the lateral malleolus distally. The proximal end lends attachment for the fibular collateral ligament of the knee and biceps femoris tendon, and the lateral malleolus forms the lateral aspect of the ankle. Provided that the head of the fibula is retained for knee stability and the distal fourth is retained for ankle stability, the body can be removed without affecting knee or ankle function. In children, however, a synostosis must be performed distally (Fig. 3-1) to prevent ankle instability.

The *medial surface of the fibular body* gives rise to the anterior muscles of the leg, the interosseous membrane (from the interosseous border), and, posterior to this membrane, the tibialis posterior muscle. The *posterior surface* gives rise to the soleus and flexor hallucis longus, while the *lateral surface* gives rise to the

peroneus longus in its proximal two thirds and peroneus brevis in its distal two thirds.

The fibula receives its *periosteal vascular supply* from the surrounding muscles, which are themselves supplied by multiple branches of the peroneal artery. The nutrient artery provides the *endosteal supply* and is also a branch of the peroneal artery. The *peroneal artery* is the largest branch of the posterior tibial artery. Near the ankle, it is connected to the posterior tibial artery by a horizontal communicating branch, and by a perforating branch to the anterior tibial artery. It arises 2–3 cm below the lower border of the popliteus and passes laterally to the fibula. Here, it lies within the substance of the flexor hallucis longus or between this muscle and the tibialis posterior in the posterior compartment of the leg. It travels just posterior to the interosseous membrane and has paired venae comitantes. The *nutrient artery* enters the fibula on the medial surface just posterior to the medial crest; this is in the middle third of the bone. It also gives off branches to surrounding muscles, but there are no other major branches in the middle two fourths of the bone. The peroneal vessels lie near the posterior tibial neurovascular bundle, separated by the tibialis posterior. No nerve accompanies the peroneal vascular bundle.

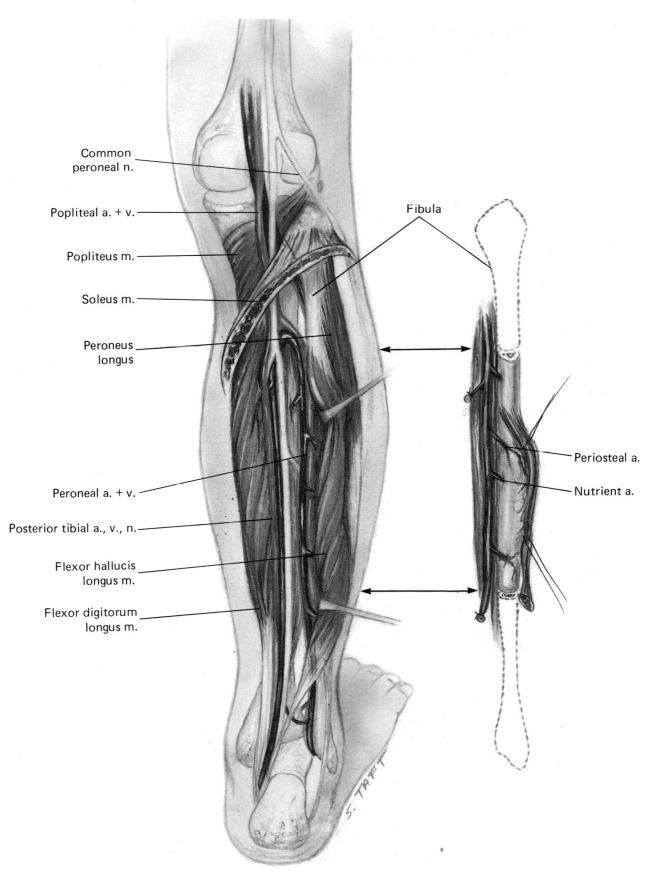

Plate 3-II. Anatomy of the vascularized fibula transplant.

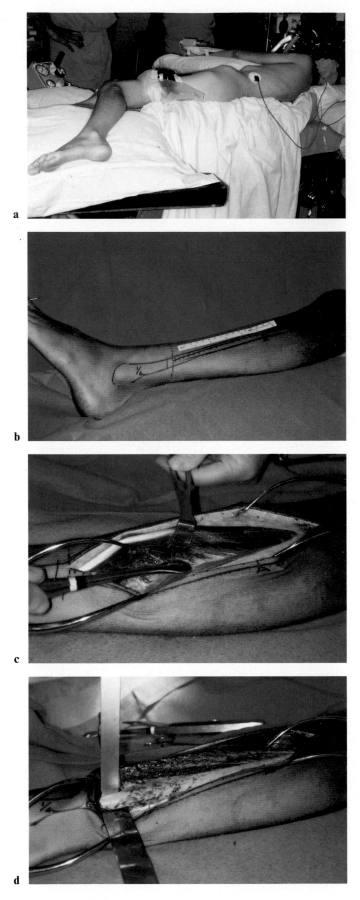

3.4.2 Surgical Technique
(Fig. 3-11; see also Fig. 3-9)

a. The leg is positioned on a well-padded arm board which extends from the operating room table. Even with the patient supine, internal rotation of the hip allows the leg to rest with the fibula uppermost.

b. The surface markings of the fibula can be seen. The distal fourth of the fibula is retained to prevent ankle instability, especially in children. The site where the peroneal nerve crosses over the neck of the fibula is noted. The length of fibula required is measured.

c. Under tourniquet control, the incision is made down to deep fascia, which is incised over the subcutaneous border of the fibula. The interval between the peroneal and soleus muscles is separated. A periosteal elevator is used to lightly remove the muscle origin from the superficial surface of the fibula. The periosteum is not removed.

d. Using an oscillating saw, the distal osteotomy is made, with care taken to protect the peroneal vessels on the deep surface of the bone.

e. With the muscle carefully retracted, the distal half of the interosseous membrane is divided.

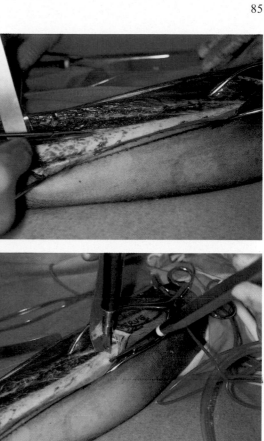

f. The proximal osteotomy is made.

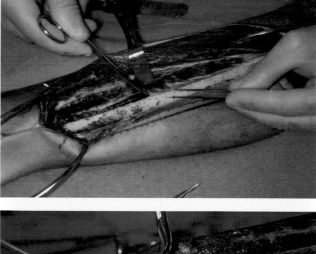

g. The fibula can now be rotated externally, bringing the interosseous membrane and the deep surface into view. The rest of the interosseous membrane is divided from the anterior aspect. Proximally, the peroneal vessels can be seen as they approach the fibula, so dissection in this region must be done cautiously. Distally, the fibula can now be grasped with a towel clip and carefully elevated, exposing the peroneal vessels lying deep to the bone in the posterior compartment.

h. These vessels are ligated distally. (They can be dissected for further length if a "flow-through" fibula transplant is planned.)

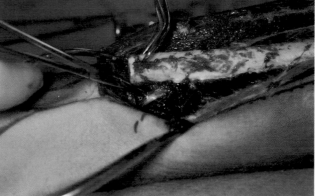

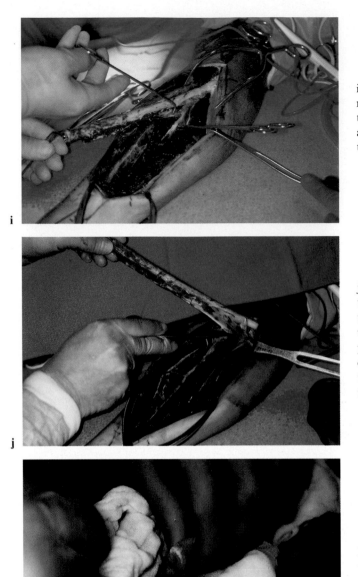

i. The fibula is now elevated, dividing deep muscle attachments but ensuring both that the peroneal vessels remain with the bone and that no communications between the vessels and bone are interrupted. (Note the proximity of the posterior tibial nerve.)

j. Proximally, the division between the peroneal vessels and the posterior tibial vessels can be identified. This division is the limit of the proximal dissection of the peroneal vessels, which are shown here. Once the recipient site has been prepared, the vascular pedicle is divided. Greater pedicle length can be obtained if less proximal fibula is required. The nutrient vessel enters the middle third of the bone, which dictates the limit of pedicle length available proximally.

k. Good bleeding from the distal medullary cavity and periosteum confirms good circulation.

l. One fourth of the fibula remains. A screw is used to accomplish the distal tibiofibular synostosis.

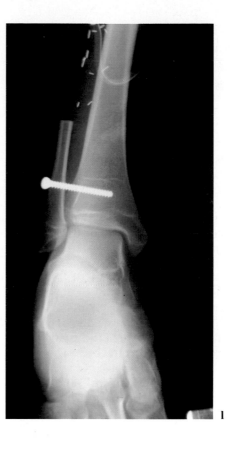

3.5 Vascularized Iliac Crest Transplantation

(Huang et al. 1980, Taylor et al. 1979, Taylor 1983, Weiland et al. 1979, Wood 1986)

3.5.1 Anatomy (Plate 3-III)

The *ilium* consists of two parts: a *body* and an *ala*. The body forms two fifths of the acetabulum. The ala is the fan-shaped, expanded portion having an inner and outer surface bounded by the *crest*. The crest is concave in its anterior part, forming the iliac fossa, but is convex behind. The crest has an overhanging external lip to which the fascia lata, external oblique muscle in its anterior half, and tensor fasciae latae muscle are attached. Attached to the internal lip are the iliac fascia and the transversus abdominis muscle. The intermediate line of the crest gives origin to the internal oblique muscle. The iliac crest ends anteriorly in the anterior superior iliac spine, to which the inguinal ligament and sartorius muscle are attached. The iliacus muscle is attached to the pelvic surface of the ala, while the gluteal muscles attach to the external surface.

Between the anterior superior iliac spine and the pubic tubercle is the inferior margin of the external oblique muscle aponeurosis, which is known as the *inguinal ligament*. The *inguinal canal*, which is about 4 cm long, lies above and parallel to the inguinal ligament. The deep inguinal ring lies above the midpoint of the inguinal ligament, while the superficial ring lies above and lateral to the pubic tubercle.

The *external iliac artery* passes under the midpoint of the inguinal ligament, and then becomes the femoral artery. The external iliac artery is crossed by the genital branch of the genitofemoral nerve and the deep circumflex iliac vein. The ductus deferens in the male and the round ligament in the female curve across its medial side. The external iliac vein lies to its medial side. The external iliac artery has two branches. The *inferior epigastric artery* emanates from its medial side just above the inguinal ligament and travels toward the umbilicus. Just lateral to the origin of this artery is the deep inguinal ring with the ductus deferens or round ligament.

The *deep circumflex iliac artery* emanates from the lateral aspect of the external iliac artery slightly distal to the inferior epigastric artery. It passes obliquely toward the anterior superior iliac spine between the transversalis fascia and the iliac fascia. It pierces the transversalis fascia and transversus abdominis to lie between the transversus abdominis and internal oblique muscles. It then passes laterally along the inside of the iliac fossa 1–2 cm from the crest. An ascending branch, frequently of considerable size, originates 1–2 cm medial to the anterior superior iliac spine. The musculocutaneous perforators travel from the deep circumflex iliac vessel to supply the overlying skin along this axis. They emerge from the external oblique muscle adjacent to the upper border of the iliac crest. The largest perforator, which is usually the continuation of the deep circumflex iliac artery, is 6–8 cm beyond the anterior superior iliac spine (Taylor et al. 1979).

Strips of the three muscles of the abdominal wall and the iliacus muscle are retained with the graft to preserve the blood supply to the bone and skin. The deep circumflex iliac vessels provide a pedicle about 6–8 cm long before entering the ilium. Its external diameter is generally 1.5-2.0 mm. The position of the deep circumflex iliac vein varies somewhat, but it can usually be located at a point 2–3 cm lateral to the external iliac artery where the artery and vein converge.

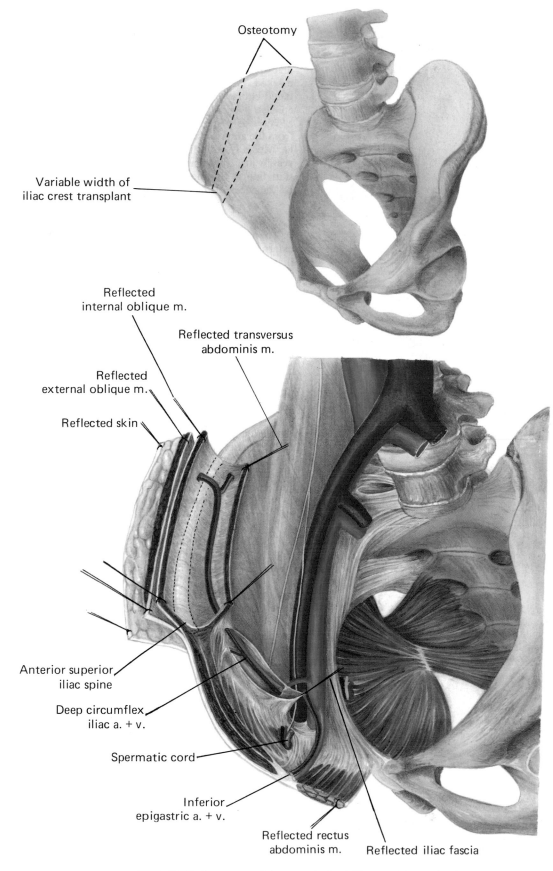

Osteotomy

Variable width of
iliac crest transplant

Reflected
internal oblique m.

Reflected transversus
abdominis m.

Reflected
external oblique m.

Reflected skin

Anterior superior
iliac spine

Deep circumflex
iliac a. + v.

Spermatic cord

Inferior
epigastric a. + v.

Reflected rectus
abdominis m.

Reflected iliac fascia

Plate 3-III. Anatomy of the vascularized iliac crest transplant.

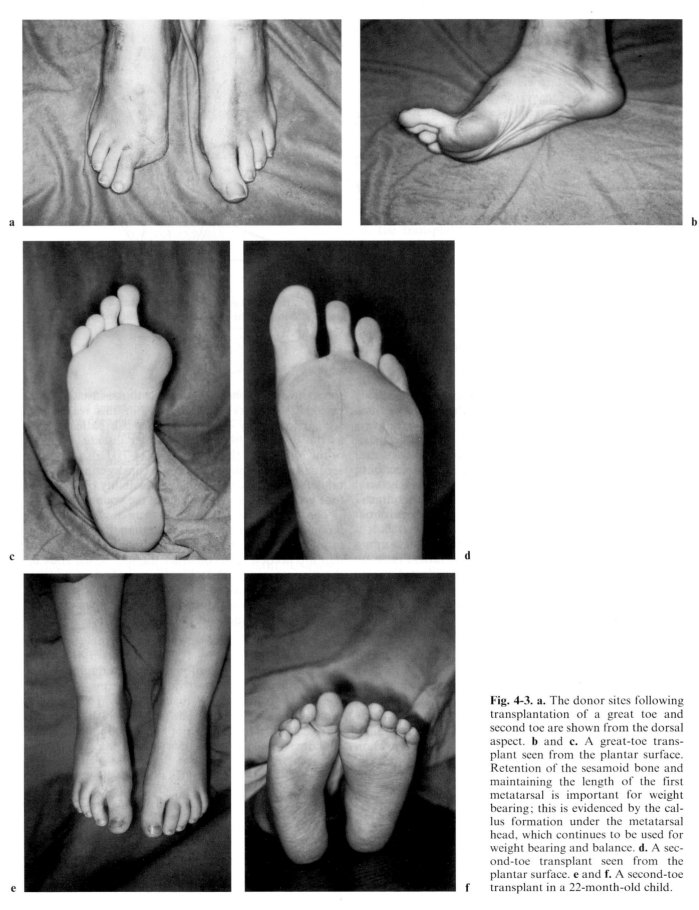

Fig. 4-3. a. The donor sites following transplantation of a great toe and second toe are shown from the dorsal aspect. **b** and **c.** A great-toe transplant seen from the plantar surface. Retention of the sesamoid bone and maintaining the length of the first metatarsal is important for weight bearing; this is evidenced by the callus formation under the metatarsal head, which continues to be used for weight bearing and balance. **d.** A second-toe transplant seen from the plantar surface. **e** and **f.** A second-toe transplant in a 22-month-old child.

4.4 Preoperative Planning

4.4.1 Arterial System

An *arteriogram of the hand* is essential in posttraumatic cases to establish which vessels are available and confirm the vascular supply to the remaining digits. The supply to the remaining digits should not be disturbed. Dominant radial supply or independent radial and ulnar supply is not infrequent (Coleman and Anson 1961, Sec. 2.9; Jones and O'Brien 1985) (Fig. 2-1). In congenital cases, the vessels are extremely small and arteriography is more difficult. It has not been my practice to perform arteriography in small children.

Because *the vascular anatomy* in the foot has considerable variability, a lateral projection arteriogram is performed to delineate the dorsal and plantar circulation (Gu et al. 1985, Leung et al. 1983, Wu et al. 1980). Spasm can be a problem in obtaining information about the distal vasculature, so vasodilating agents or a general anesthetic may sometimes be indicated when doing the arteriogram. The position of the first dorsal metatarsal artery, i.e., dorsal or plantar, may be seen on an oblique arteriogram of the foot. Also, if this artery curves under the first metatarsal on the anteroposterior view, a plantar vessel can be anticipated. A detailed knowledge of the vascular anatomy of the first metatarsal artery is the key to the arterial dissection for both second- and great-toe transplantation (Leung et al. 1980, Wu et al. 1980) (Plates 4-III and 4-V; Fig. 1-23c).

4.4.2 Venous System

The veins should be outlined on the *dorsum of the foot* by elevating the tourniquet so that blood pressure is between systolic and diastolic. The veins on the *dorsal aspect of the hand* forming the dorsal venous network drain into the basilic and cephalic veins; these are of large caliber and make excellent recipient vessels. After a burn, or if there has been extensive skin grafting on the dorsal aspect of the hand, these vessels may be absent, in which case the venae comitantes of the radial artery should be used.

4.4.3 Osteosynthesis

Length is a key factor for both appearance and function of the transplanted toe. A reconstructed thumb or finger that is slightly shorter than its contralateral counterpart will generally function well. When planning length, the arcade of the digits must be kept in mind. One should also be aware that the method of bone fixation will affect the ultimate length and should therefore be planned carefully. Bone fixation can be accomplished with (1) the end-to-end technique, using Kirschner wires or interosseous wires (Fig. 5-24), or (2) the overlapping technique, wherein the toe bone is hollowed out and a peg is fashioned on the thumb. This creates a mortise-and-tenon joint with good bone contact, and it is secured with a single oblique Kirschner wire to control rotation.

4.4.4 Skin Flaps

Skin flaps, transplant length, and the position of the vascular pedicle can be planned with a *clay model* (Figs. 4-8, 4-16, and 4-19). For example, if the first web space has poor soft-tissue cover, as large a skin flap as possible should be taken with the toe.

When the ipsilateral toe is used, the skin on the lateral aspect of the great toe and the first toe web space can be included to provide cover or release a contracture of the first web space in the hand. In addition, the arterial pedicle will then be in the correct position to anastomose the dorsalis pedis vessel to the radial artery just before this artery enters between the two heads of the first dorsal interosseous muscle. When fingers are being reconstructed, the webs and position of the vessels should be planned similarly.

The *web space of the toe* lies at the mid-proximal phalanx level of the toes. If the osteotomy site of the toe transplant is more proximal, skin cover proximal to this level will be inadequate and either a split-thickness skin graft or another method of skin cover will be necessary (Fig. 4-1).

Any first *web space contracture* should be released; this can be accomplished with coronal incisions over the thumb amputation stump with flap elevation on the radial and ulnar sides, which should allow for the skin on the ulnar aspect of the amputation stump to drop into the first web space. If this measure is anticipated to be inadequate, a preliminary procedure to provide adequate soft-tissue coverage may be necessary prior to toe-to-thumb transplantation.

In deciding whether to use the *left or right great toe*, one must consider (1) that the ipsilateral toe taken with some skin from the first web space will provide better cover for the first web space of the hand; (2) that the ipsilateral great toe will be angled about 10° toward the index finger at the interphalangeal joint and may compromise large object grasp slightly (May et al. 1978); and (3) the position of the arteries. Transplanting the ipsilateral toe will place the dorsalis pedis vessel close to the radial artery as this artery enters between the two heads of the first dorsal interosseous muscle.

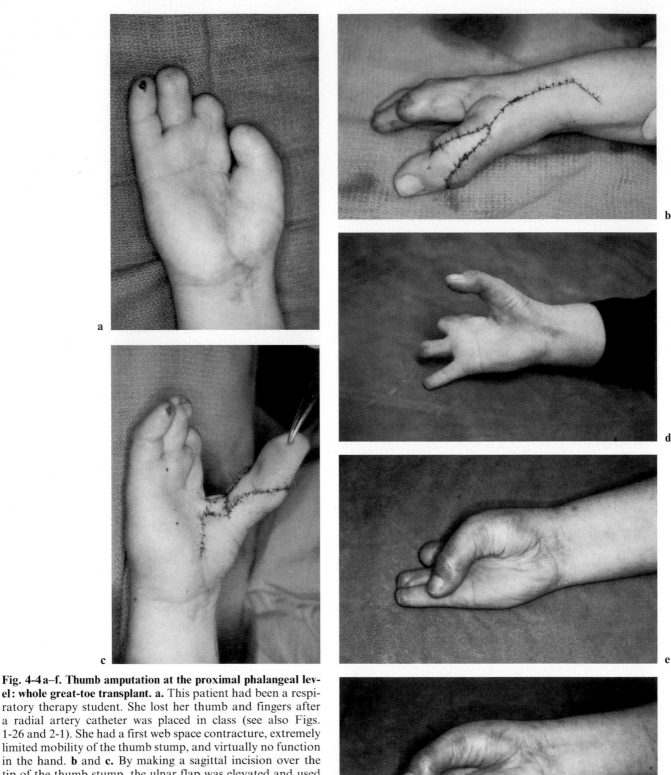

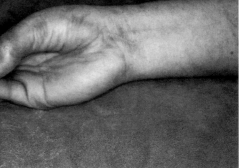

Fig. 4-4a–f. Thumb amputation at the proximal phalangeal level: whole great-toe transplant. a. This patient had been a respiratory therapy student. She lost her thumb and fingers after a radial artery catheter was placed in class (see also Figs. 1-26 and 2-1). She had a first web space contracture, extremely limited mobility of the thumb stump, and virtually no function in the hand. **b** and **c.** By making a sagittal incision over the tip of the thumb stump, the ulnar flap was elevated and used to widen the first web space. The thumb was then planned with flaps to fit appropriately over the end of the bone. With the ulnar artery being the dominant vessel supplying this patient's hand, the arterial anastomosis was performed between the dorsalis pedis vessel and the radial artery proximal to the wrist. **d–f.** The transplant looks very similar to a thumb. The patient is able to pinch against the small finger and has regained both large and small object grasp.

Fig. 4-5a–e. Thumb amputation at the distal metacarpal level: whole great-toe transplant. a. The great toe appears slightly broader than the thumb when the two are seen next to each other. When seen separately, the appearance is good. **b.** Especially if there is no movement in the metacarpophalangeal joint, a functional interphalangeal joint is important. Fifteen to 30° of motion can usually be achieved (Frykman et al. 1986). **c** and **d.** Good dexterity and large object grasp were restored. **e.** Seven-millimeter two-point discrimination (Frykman et al. 1986).

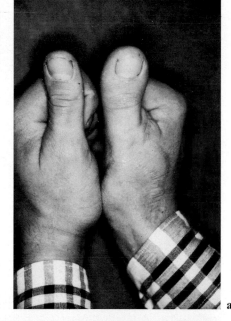

a

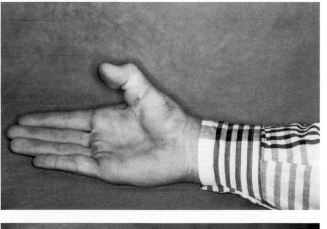

b

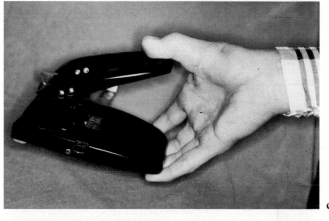

c

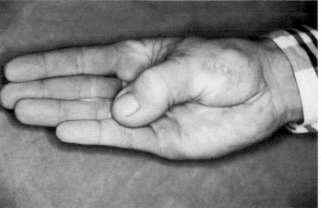

d

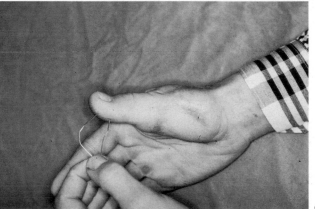

e

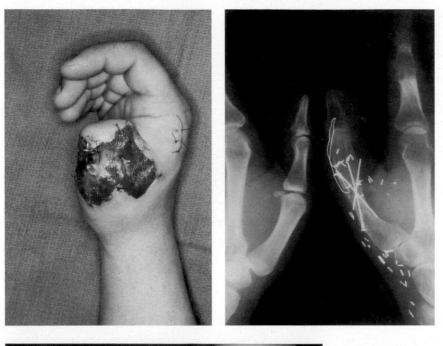

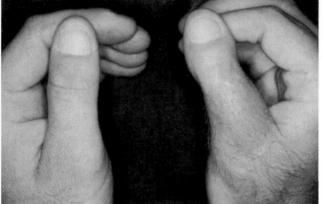

Fig. 4-6a–c. Thumb amputation at the distal metacarpal level: "wrap-around" procedure (see also Fig. 4-21). **a.** A 22-year-old man sustained a thumb amputation with a crush injury of the distal metacarpal. A tubed groin flap was used preliminarily to provide soft-tissue cover in anticipation of a toe wrap-around procedure. **b.** An iliac crest corticocancellous graft was wired to the distal metacarpal. The distal aspect of this iliac crest graft was fixed to the distal phalanx of the toe transplant. **c.** A thumb was reconstructed which had an excellent appearance and good function. The only movement possible is at the carpometacarpal joint. (Courtesy of Hill Hastings II, M.D.)

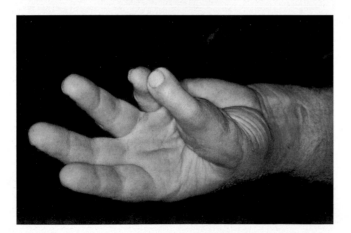

Fig. 4-7. Thumb amputation in a high-risk patient: second toe-to-thumb transplant. This patient has polycythemia. He chose to undergo second-toe transplantation because the appearance of the donor site is better than that of any other transplant; this was an important consideration because I felt he had a slightly greater risk of losing the transplant. This transplant is considerably narrower than a normal thumb or a thumb reconstructed from either a great toe or by the wrap-around procedure. It is flexed at the interphalangeal joint and has the appearance of a toe. Despite the transplant's narrower pulp surface and lesser strength compared with a transplanted great toe, this patient regained adequate function and was satisfied with the result.

Fig. 4-8 a–h. Thumb amputation at the trapezium level: second-toe ray transplant including the second metatarsal. a. In an accident involving an auger, this man's thumb was amputated at the trapezium level. There were severe injuries to all of the other fingers, partial amputation of the ring and small fingers, and nerve and tendon damage to the index and long fingers. **b.** A second-toe transplant including the second metatarsal was planned to provide some opposition. Because of severe injuries to the radial aspect of the hand, the index finger had poor sensation on the radial side. This deficit in addition to the injuries to the other digits made pollicization a less desirable alternative. **c.** Following the toe transplant, an *adduction contracture* was present in the first web space, and the thumb had no *active opposition*. A flap was needed in the first web space to release the contracture, and active motor function was required to enable opposition and thumb abduction. A Huber abductor digiti minimi transfer was considered as an active motor, but additional tissue was needed to allow passive motion in the web space. A serratus muscle transplant satisfied both of these requirements simultaneously. The web space was released and the recurrent branch of the median nerve was dissected and divided proximal to the neuroma for repair to the long thoracic nerve fascicles. **d.** One slip of the serratus anterior was used to widen the web space, and a second slip brought subcutaneously to the radial aspect of the thumb provided abduction. **e.** This muscle transplant released the first web space contracture and restored good active abduction and opposition. The muscle is flat and profiles evenly with the surrounding palmar skin. The similarity between the actual reconstruction and the clay model is evident. (*Continued*)

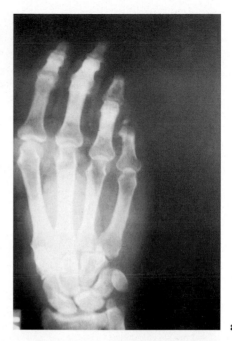

a

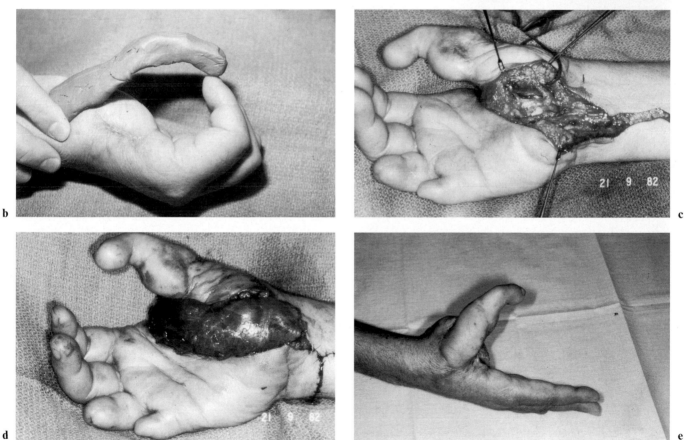

b

c

d

e

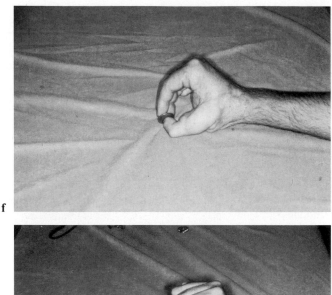

f

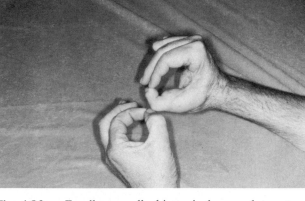

g

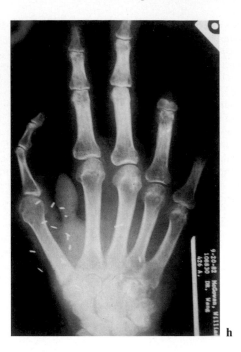

h

Fig. 4-8 f, g. Excellent small object pinch was also restored with reasonable appearance of the thumb, as shown here. The interphalangeal joint remains flexed, which is a frequent occurrence following second-toe transplantation to either the finger or thumb position. **h.** Initially, the metacarpal was pinned to the trapezium. When the pin was removed after 4 months, a "pseudo-arthrosis" formed between the base of the metacarpal and the trapezium. Movement at this joint was confirmed by fluoroscopy. The patient has no pain or discomfort during movement. He fully resumed work as a butcher without problems or limitations.

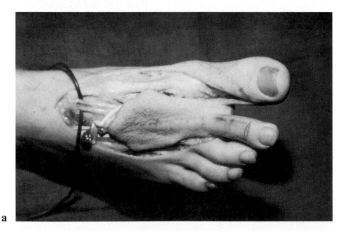

a

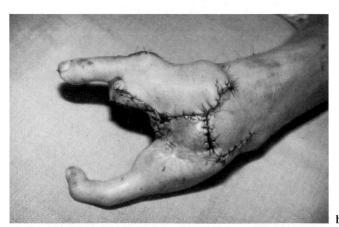

b

Fig. 4-9 a, b. Thumb amputation at the base of the metacarpal: second-toe ray transplant with a dorsalis pedis flap. a. When the second-toe ray including the metatarsal is transplanted, the sides of the metatarsal need soft-tissue cover, although the interosseous muscle may cover a part of this area. The cover options are (1) a preliminary cutaneous flap, (2) a split-thickness skin graft on the muscle tissue, (3) a dorsalis pedis flap taken with the toe transplant, and (4) a flap done at the time of the toe transplant. If a dorsalis pedis flap is taken, skin grafting will be required after removing the second-toe ray. This grafting is a disadvantage because it can lead to delayed healing in the foot. Here, a dorsalis pedis flap with the second toe is seen dissected. Proximally, the vessels and extensor tendon have been dissected. **b.** This second-toe transplant was used in the thumb position to provide opposition against a stiff small finger. The flap was well vascularized, but additional skin grafting was required on the palmar surface.

Fig. 4-10a–f. Thumb agenesis: second-toe to thumb transplant. a. This 22-month-old girl had bilateral symmetrical congenital hand deformities, with a rudimentary thumb and two poorly functioning digits. A thumb for opposition was needed. In such a deficiency, it is necessary to first dissect the vessels, nerves, and tendons in the hand to assess whether recipient structures are present and toe transplantation will be worthwhile. **b.** The toe was dissected. The dorsalis pedis vessel, digital nerves, and tendons were ready to be divided at the point affording the appropriate length. **c.** The improvement in the hand was compared with the opposite side. The cosmetic and functional deficit in the foot is minimal (Fig. 4-3). **d.** Large object grasp has been provided. **e.** Good, passive motion and excellent sensation is present in the transplant. Further reconstruction to provide pulp-to-pulp pinch is planned when the child is older. **f.** Solid healing of the transplant to the metacarpal is evident.

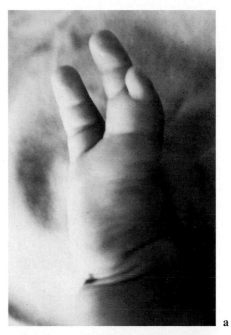

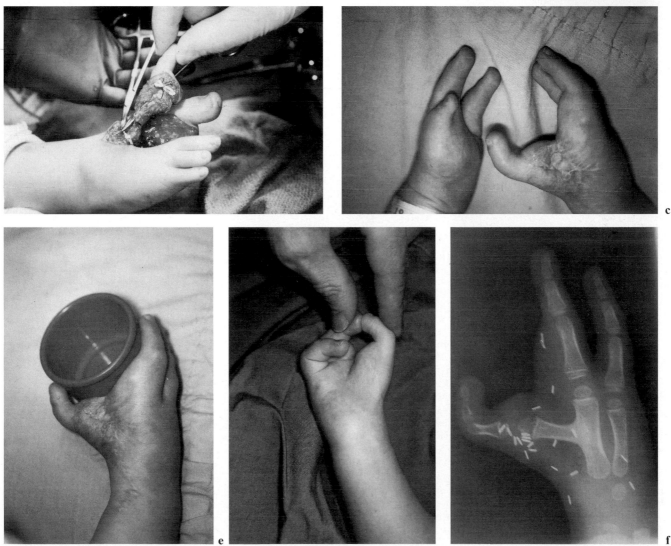

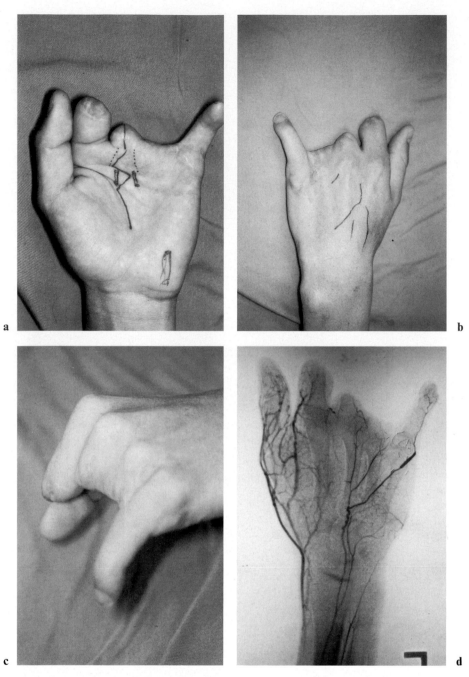

Fig. 4-11 a–j. Multiple finger amputation distal to the metacar-pophalangeal joint (one finger remaining): second-toe transplant (see also Fig. 4-22). **a.** Following a saw injury, this patient had had one finger replanted which became insensate and stiff. On the palmar surface, a second toe was to be transferred to the long finger position to restore pinch and provide a broader surface for tubular and large object grasp. A longitudinal incision over the tip of the long finger amputation stump opened the digit, permitting easy positioning of the toe transplant and bone fixation. The anticipated position of the digital nerves and position of the common digital vessels heard on Doppler examination were marked out on the hand. **b.** On the dorsal surface, the superficial veins were mapped out. **c.** Good flexion and extension of the metacarpophalangeal joints

were present in the fingers. This feature is extremely important for the ultimate functioning of this transplant. **d.** The preoperative arteriogram revealed separate arterial supply to the ulnar and radial parts of the hand (see also Figs. 1-26 and 2-1). It is essential in this situation to use a digital vessel or the radial artery end-to-side. **e.** Dissection of the palmar structures revealed a good digital artery, common digital nerve, and flexor tendons. **f.** On the dorsal side, a long vein was harvested with the toe for anastomosis to the dorsal venous system of the hand. **g–j.** A broad surface has been established for grasp of large objects. The patient uses the transplant for pinch and manipulation of small objects and for key pinch and other activities requiring strength.

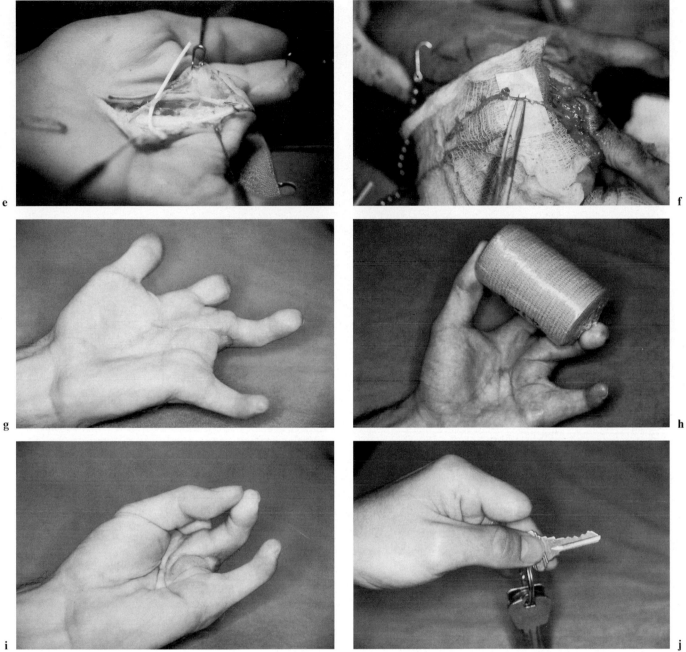

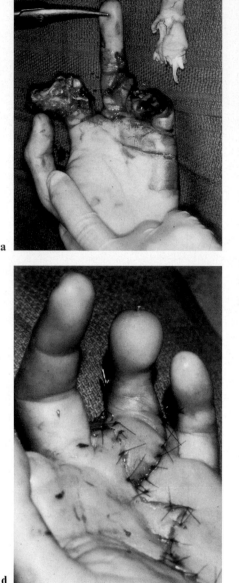

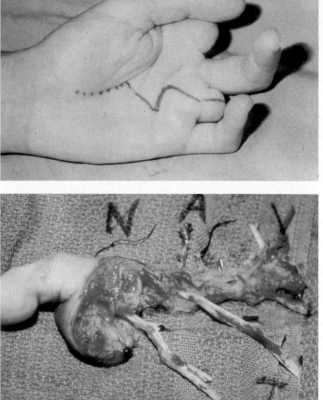

Fig. 4-12a–d. Multiple finger amputation distal to the metacarpophalangeal joint (two fingers remaining): second-toe transplant. a. A 30-year-old woman sustained severe injuries to all of her digits in a saw accident. b. The long finger regained reasonable function following repair, but sensation was impaired and movement was poor. The small finger was stiff and had limited function. The incision was marked out. c. A second toe was harvested for transplantation; the structures are shown. d. The toe was transplanted to the ring finger position, restoring the arcade of the digits and markedly improving the appearance of the hand. The interphalangeal joint of the toe was pinned to avoid the distinctly flexed attitude of this joint. (Ultimate function of a toe transplanted to the finger position largely depends on mobility at the metacarpophalangeal joint because the interphalangeal joints cannot be expected to regain good flexion and extension. Good sensation, however, is usually restored.)

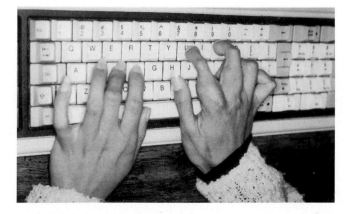

Fig. 4-13. Multiple finger amputation distal to the metacarpophalangeal joint (normal ring and small fingers): double second-toe transplant. This patient sustained an amputation of the index and long fingers and was unable to work as a typist. She was also particularly distressed by the appearance of her hand. Despite the use of a cosmetic prosthesis, she continued to have problems and was unable to work. A double second-toe transplant (one toe from each foot) restored the normal arcade of the digits. Although these digits have the appearance of toes on close scrutiny – being in a flexed position at the interphalangeal joints – the patient indicated that this is never noticed and she is exceedingly pleased with the result. She is once again able to work as a typist. Toe transplantation may be indicated in such unusual circumstances where five-fingered activities and cosmetic considerations are important.

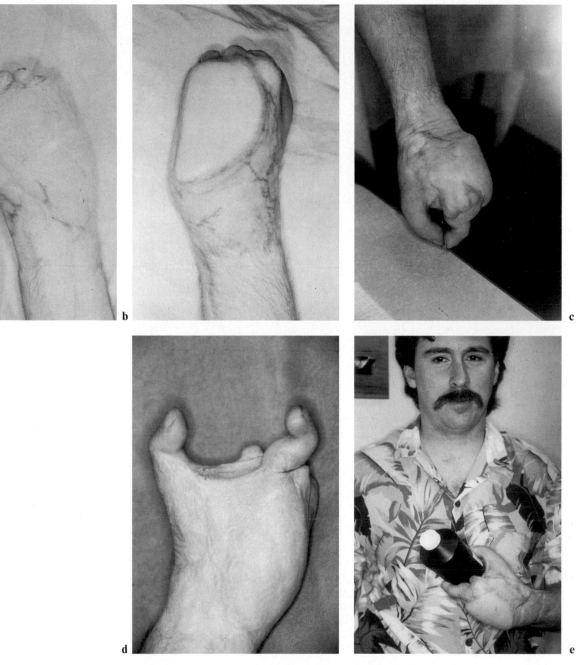

Fig. 4-14a–e. Adactyly with an intact thumb (traumatic): second-toe transplant (see also Fig. 1-8). **a** and **b.** This patient sustained an exceedingly severe crush injury to his hand. A double microvascular muscle transplant provided cover, with the latissimus dorsi used dorsally and the serratus anterior placed on the palmar surface (Fig. 1-8). His thumb had good sensation and some motion, but a mobile digit was needed on the ulnar side to provide pinch. In a preliminary operation, silicone tendon rods were placed under the muscle transplant on the palmar and dorsal sides to provide gliding surfaces for the flexor and extensor tendons of the proposed toe transplant. **c–e.** The patient regained excellent large and small object grasp. There was good movement and sensation in the finger with good end-to-end pinch.

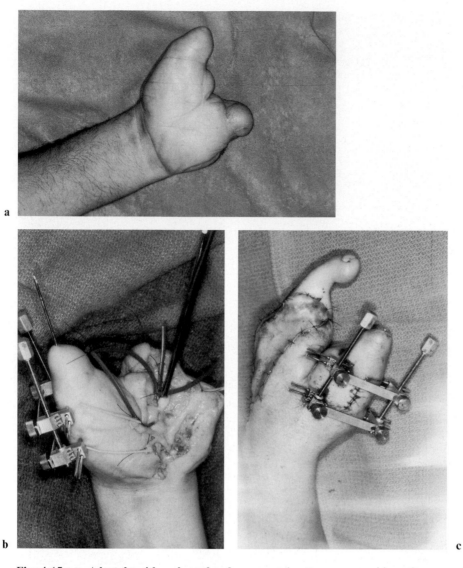

Fig. 4-15a–c. Adactyly with a short thumb remnant (posttraumatic): second-toe transplantation combined with thumb lengthening. a. Reconstruction of this hand required a new digit on the ulnar side as well as adequate thumb length for opposition. The option of double toe transplantation was considered, but because the thenar muscles were still functional and could provide active opposition, thumb lengthening was chosen. **b.** The lengthening apparatus was placed on the thumb metacarpal. The recipient structures were dissected to receive the second-toe transplant. **c.** The second-toe transplant is seen in place. Note that a skin graft was needed to cover the dorsal aspect of the second metatarsal.

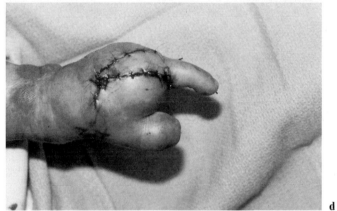

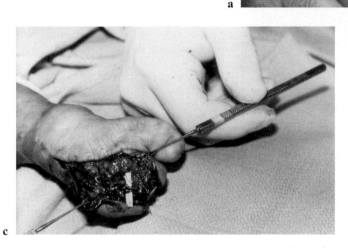

Fig. 4-16a–d. Congenital multiple finger loss: transplant of a second toe to the long finger position. a and **b.** Congenital amputation of the fingers left this 3-year-old boy with only a short thumb in his left hand. A second-toe transplant was planned to provide a mobile, opposing digit. A clay model was used to plan the position of the vascular repairs and skin flaps, and the length, position, and rotation of the trans- plant on the hand. **c.** The vessels and nerves were present near the site of amputation. **d.** The toe in position on the hand resembles the clay model. At the time of foot closure, an extra segment of the second metatarsal was taken. It was anticipated that this bone would be used for later thumb lengthening.

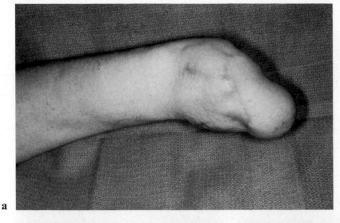

Fig. 4-17 a–c. Mitten hand (posttraumatic): great-toe and second-toe transplant. a. This 42-year-old chemist lost all of his fingers and thumb in a laboratory explosion. b. A great toe from one foot was used to reconstruct a thumb, and a second toe from the opposite foot was used to fashion an opposable digit; this restored reasonable grasp. c. Although there is no strong pulp-to-pulp pinch, pinch is possible between the thumb and index finger if he uses a broad-barrel pen.

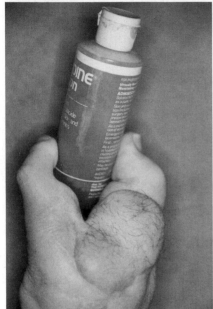

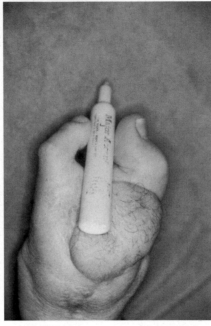

Fig. 4-18 a–c. Mitten hand (posttraumatic): great-toe transplant combined with an orthosis. a. This patient required reconstruction for an amputation at the distal metacarpal level. b and c. A great toe was used to reconstruct a thumb, and an orthosis was then used to enable pinch. An orthosis is not nearly as effective as a sensate second toe, but it is a reasonable alternative in some situations. (Courtesy of Richard J. Smith, MD†)

† Deceased.   ▽

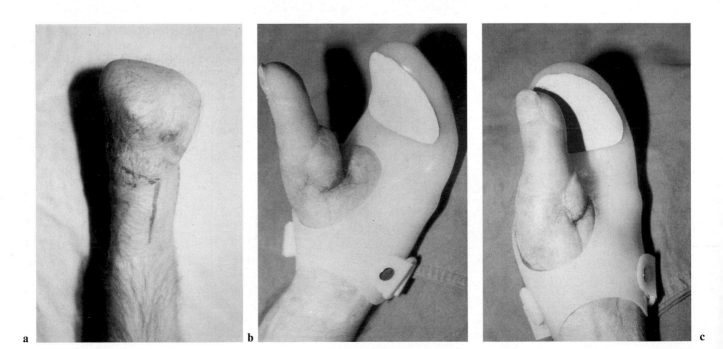

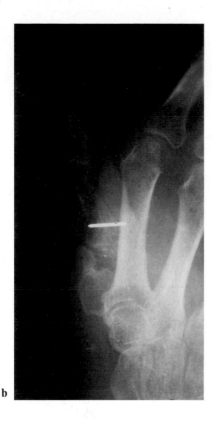

b

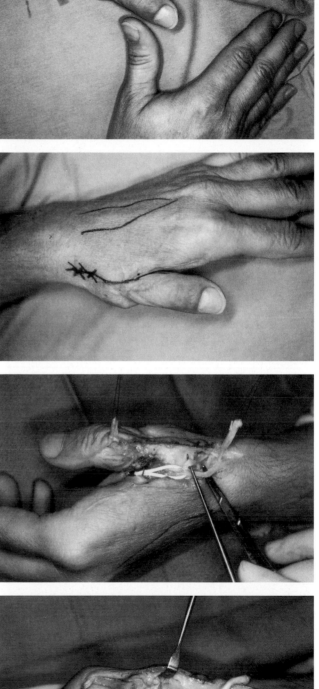

a

c

d

e

Fig. 4-19a–j. Metacarpal and metacarpophalangeal joint loss in the thumb (posttraumatic): metatarsophalangeal joint of the second toe to the thumb metacarpophalangeal joint (see also Fig. 4-24). **a.** This patient injured his right thumb in a rifle accident. There was a marked web space contracture with no passive movement. The reconstruction option chosen was to graft bone to lengthen the thumb, and release the web space contracture. This release would require a substantial amount of tissue. The bone transplant would have to include a joint because the trapeziometacarpal joint provided the only mobility. **b.** This radiograph shows the damage, which included loss of the metacarpal and metacarpophalangeal joints and marked shortening. **c.** A web space release was planned. The radial artery could be palpated on the dorsal surface of the first metacarpal space. The dorsal veins are seen outlined. **d.** The extensor tendons were dissected proximally and distally, and the radial artery is shown just before it enters between the two heads of the first dorsal interosseous muscle. A large superficial vein is also shown. **e.** The osteotomy prepared the site for the vascularized joint transplant. *Continued*

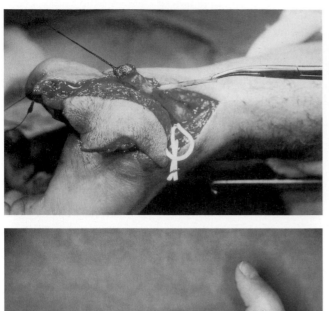

f

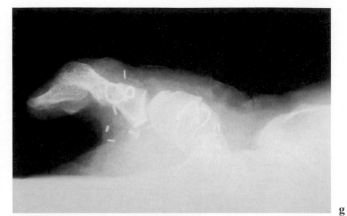

g

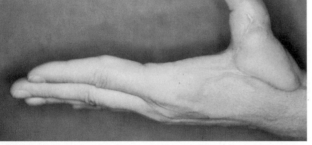

h

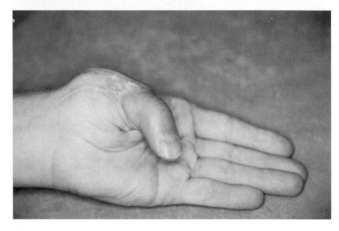

i

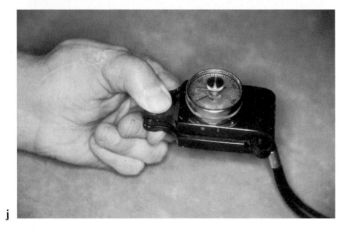

j

Fig. 4-19. f. The joint was wired into place and a weave stitch was used to repair the extensor tendons. Note that the cutaneous flap was carefully planned to provide soft-tissue cover in the first web space for abduction of the thumb. **g.** This radiograph shows the position of the joint transplant and the intraosseous wiring, which provided good fixation both proximally and distally. **h–j.** Good thumb length was restored. The patient is able to abduct well and can flex the thumb to a point 1 cm from the base of the small finger. He has good pinch strength between the thumb and index finger.

4.5 Anatomy (Plate 4-IV)

The great and second toes are hyperextended at the metatarsophalangeal joint, slightly flexed at the proximal interphalangeal joint, and extended at the distal interphalangeal joint (Plate 4-I). The longitudinal arch of the foot ends at the metatarsal head, which bears the weight of the body during gait. This overall structure differs from that of fingers, which have a longitudinally flexed arch that terminates at their end. Both the joint surfaces and joint capsules are adapted to their positions. The web spaces of the foot are located more distally than those of the hand (Fig. 4-1).

The *superficial transverse metatarsal ligaments* reinforce and connect the digital slips of the plantar aponeurosis. The articular capsule of the metatarsophalangeal joint is loose. Dorsally, it is reinforced by fibers from the extensor tendons and is attached closer to the articular border than it is on the plantar side. The *plantar ligament* is analogous to the palmar plate of the fingers. On each side of the joint lies a collateral ligament. The plantar ligament of the great toe is replaced by the sesamoid bones and a strong interconnecting ligament between them. All of the plantar ligaments are connected by *deep transverse metatarsal ligaments* which connect adjacent metatarsal heads and joint capsules.

At ankle level, the *anterior tibial artery* lies between the extensor hallucis longus and extensor digitorum longus tendons. At the ankle it becomes the *dorsalis pedis artery* which passes over the dorsum of the foot to the first intermetatarsal space. Just proximal to this space, it is crossed by the extensor hallucis brevis tendon, and at the base it divides into the *deep plantar artery* (also called the perforating branch), which dives plantarward to the plantar arch, and the *first dorsal metatarsal artery*, which proceeds distally in the first metatarsal space. Distally, this vessel divides into two branches which supply the adjacent sides of the first web space.

The *origin of the first dorsal metatarsal artery is of considerable surgical importance* and can be somewhat variable (Plate 4-V). In about two thirds of patients, the first dorsal metatarsal artery emanates from the dorsalis pedis artery and travels in a relatively dorsal plane (Plate 4-VA and B). This course can be dorsal to the interosseous muscle (Plate 4-VA), within the muscle, or deep to it (Plate 4-VB), but the artery courses dorsal to the deep transverse metatarsal ligament (Plate 4-VA and B). Other configurations are seen in about one third of patients. The first dorsal metatarsal may arise from the dorsalis pedis or deep plantar artery, but the principal vessel to the toes runs deep to the deep transverse metatarsal ligament (Plate 4-VC). Occasionally, the vessels to the great and second toes may arise from the plantar arterial arch (Plate 4–VD) (Egloff 1984, Leung et al. 1983).

The dorsalis pedis artery has paired *venae comitantes*.

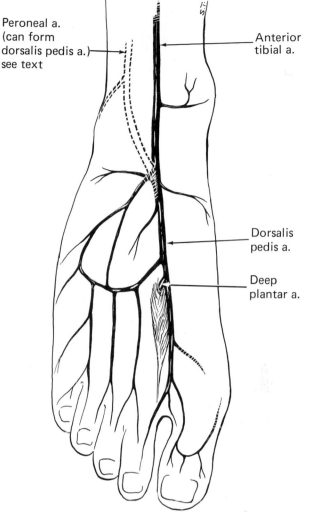

Plate 4-III. The dorsalis pedis artery can arise from the peroneal artery on the lateral aspect of the ankle (see also Fig. 1-23c).

Superficial veins on the dorsum of the foot form a venous arch and drain into the saphenous system.

The *deep peroneal nerve* divides just distal to the ankle into medial and lateral branches. The medial branch passes distally just lateral or medial to the dorsalis pedis artery and divides into two dorsal digital nerves which supply the *adjacent sides of the first web space* (Fig. 2-12c). The *superficial peroneal nerve* pierces the deep fascia proximal to the ankle between the peroneus longus and extensor digitorum longus, and divides into two branches. The medial and intermediate dorsal cutaneous nerves cross the ankle to supply the *dorsum of the foot* (Fig. 2-12b), while the nerve supply to the *plantar surfaces* of the medial 3 1/2 toes arises from the *medial plantar nerve*. The medial plantar nerve gives off the proper digital nerve to the great toe, and three common digital nerves which pass between the divisions of the plantar aponeurosis; these common digital nerves divide into proper digital nerves which pass plantar to the digital arteries along both sides of each toe.

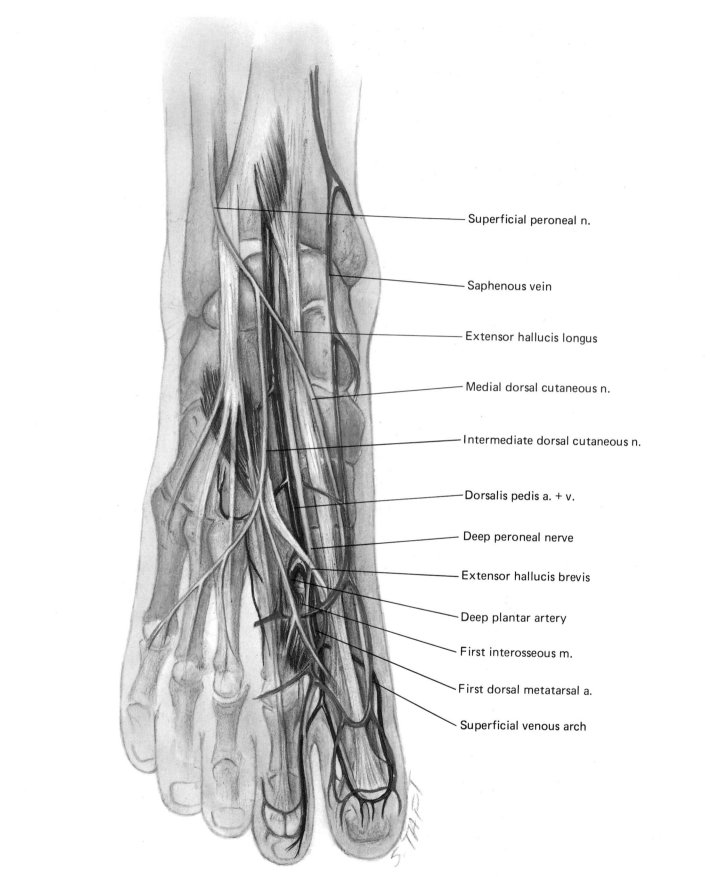

— Superficial peroneal n.

— Saphenous vein

— Extensor hallucis longus

— Medial dorsal cutaneous n.

— Intermediate dorsal cutaneous n.

— Dorsalis pedis a. + v.

— Deep peroneal nerve

— Extensor hallucis brevis

— Deep plantar artery

— First interosseous m.

— First dorsal metatarsal a.

— Superficial venous arch

Plate 4-IV. Anatomy of the dorsum of the foot.

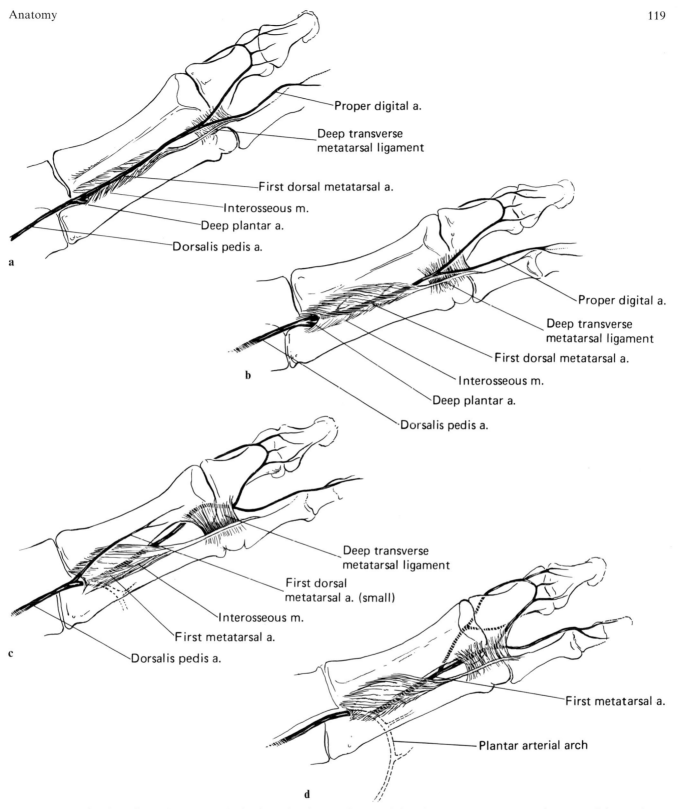

Plate 4-V. a. The dorsalis pedis artery divides into the deep plantar artery and the first dorsal metatarsal artery (FDMA). The FDMA continues superficial to the interosseous muscle and deep transverse metatarsal ligament, and divides into the proper digital arteries supplying the adjacent sides of the first web space. **b.** The FDMA can travel in or deep to the interosseous muscle, but remains superficial to the deep transverse metatarsal ligament. **c.** The FDMA is small and inadequate for supplying the toes. The metatarsal artery originates from the dorsalis pedis artery or the deep plantar artery, and runs deep to the interosseous muscle and deep transverse metatarsal ligament. This artery tends to curve under the first metatarsal bone. **d.** The first metatarsal artery emanates from the plantar arterial arch and runs deep to the interosseous muscle and deep transverse metatarsal ligament. The FDMA is small or absent.

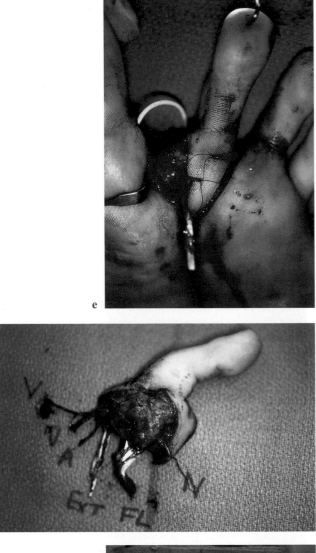

e

f

g

e. On the plantar surface, the *flexor tendon* is dissected and divided (Fig. 4-20 h). The *digital nerves* are dissected and tagged with 6-0 silk for later retrieval.

f. In this patient, the *toe* was removed and the capsule was divided at the metatarsophalangeal joint. The structures are shown.

g. During the hand dissection, the required length of each structure should be recorded.

The toe is transferred to the *hand*. Various methods of osteosynthesis may be used (Sec. 4.4). With the distal interphalangeal joint in extension, a Kirschner wire is placed across the joint to avoid the problem of excessive flexion of the second-toe transplant. This wire is removed 2–3 weeks later. Tendon repairs are performed using a Pulvertaft weave stitch. This tenorrhaphy is strong enough to allow early range of motion. If possible, any pulleys in the A1 or A2 region proximal to the transplant should be retained because they will optimize ultimate motion. The nerves are then repaired using 9-0 nylon suture without tension.

4.6.3.1 Foot Closure

After second-toe or second metatarsophalangeal joint transplantation, ray amputation of the second toe usually produces the best functional and cosmetic result. The second metatarsal is divided back at the base, and the first and third metatarsals are approximated. A strong repair of the intermetatarsal ligament between these metatarsals is done, ensuring proper position, spacing, and rotation. Temporary Kirschner wires may be helpful, and routine skin closure without tension completes the repair.

4.6.4 Partial Toe Transplantation
(Foucher et al. 1980) (Fig. 4-23)

While various parts of the great or second toe can be used to reconstruct fingers, the procedure must be tailored to the specific needs of the injured digit. The distal phalanx along with its soft tissues, or soft tissue alone can be carried on the vascular pedicle. Either surface, plantar or dorsal, can be transplanted separately. The lateral half of the great toe and medial half of the second toe can be used as neurovascular transplants to resurface the palm or digits. This transplant can include a skin flap from the dorsum of the foot, making it a Y-shaped flap.

The sensory potential of such a flap is similar to that of skin following digital nerve repair. One can expect a good functional result because untraumatized

nerve is sutured without any tension (Lipton et al. 1987, Poppen et al. 1983). This method enables reconstruction of the distal palm and adjacent web spaces of the fingers, and parts of the pulp of the fingers or thumb can be resurfaced with sensate skin. The donor site can usually be closed primarily, and the defect on the foot is slight. While many applications of this method exist, the following case is presented as a simple example.

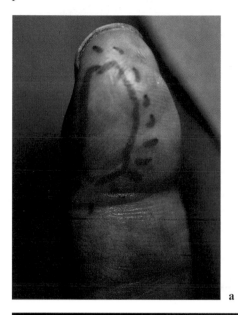

a. A 55-year-old man sustained a mangled laceration of the radial aspect of the distal phalanx of his index finger. An exquisitely tender neuroma resulted and a local flap failed to improve the condition. The neuroma was divided more proximally but the pain continued. He was referred to my care, unable to use the digit because of the severe pain. Although advised to undergo amputation, he strongly objected. Resurfacing of the sensitive distal pulp and nerve repair were planned as an alternative.

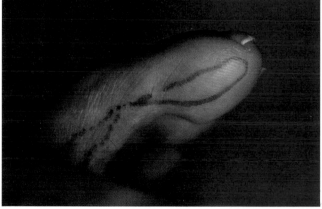

b. A neurovascular flap is outlined on the medial aspect of the second toe.

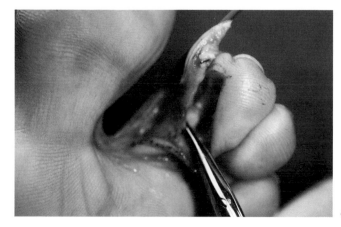

c. Under tourniquet control, the flap is elevated and the digital neurovascular bundle is dissected back to the base of the toe. This dissection includes a superficial vein.

May JW, Smith RJ, Peimer CA (1981) Toe-to-hand free tissue transfer for thumb construction with multiple digit aplasia. Plast Reconstr Surg 67:205

Meals RA, Lesavoy MA (1983) Hallux to thumb transplant during ankle disarticulation for multiple limb anomalies. JAMA 249:72

Michon J, Merle M, Bouchon Y, et al (1984) Functional comparison between pollicization and toe-to-hand transfer for thumb reconstruction. J Reconstr Microsurg 1:103

Morrison WA, O'Brien B McC, MacLeod AM (1980) Thumb reconstruction with a free neurovascular wrap-around flap from the big toe. J Hand Surg 5:575

O'Brien BM, Gould JS, Morrison WA (1984) Free vascularized small joint transfer in the hand. J Hand Surg 9A:634

O'Brien B, MacLeod AM, Sykes PJ (1978) Microvascular second toe transfer for digital reconstruction. J Hand Surg 3:123

Poppen NK, Mann RA, O'Konski M, et al (1981) Amputation of the great toe. Foot Ankle 1:333

Poppen NK, Norris TR, Buncke HJ (1983) Evaluation of sensibility and function with microsurgical free tissue transfer of the great toe to the hand for thumb reconstruction. J Hand Surg 8:516

Tsai TM, Jupiter JB, Kutz JE, et al (1982) Vascularized autogenous whole joint transfer in the hand. J Hand Surg 7:335

Wei W (1983) Keys to successful second toe-to-hand transfer. A review of 30 cases. J Hand Surg 8:902

Wilson CS, Buncke HJ, Alpert BS, Gordon L (1984) Composite metacarpophalangeal joint reconstruction in great toe-to-hand free tissue transfers. J Hand Surg 9A:645

Wray RC, Mathes SM, Young VL, et al (1981) Free vascularized whole joint transplants with ununited epiphyses. Plast Reconstr Surg 67:519

The indications for using the great toe to construct an opposable thumb in multiple digital aplasia is described. This article covers preoperative planning and surgical technique.

This is a case report of a 10-year-old boy with four anomalous limbs who had his left great toe transplanted to the left hand for use as a thumb. Simultaneously, he underwent an ankle disarticulation to improve his lower extremity function. While no active motion was achieved in the thumb, three-point grasp of light-weight objects was possible after surgery.

This retrospective study comparing pollicization with great- or second-toe transplantation for various hand defects has important practical implications. For patients who were missing the thumb but had four normal fingers, pollicization provided the best sensibility and mobility. Power was better after great-toe transplantation than after pollicization or second-toe transplantation. Pollicization in cases of relatively greater loss depended on the mobility of the proximal interphalangeal joint, the sensibility of the transferred digit, and the quality of the nontransferred digits.

The technique of placing an iliac crest bone graft to lengthen the amputated thumb and then covering this graft with a wrap-around flap of soft tissues from the great toe is presented along with five case summaries.

Seven patients, including four children, underwent vascularized joint transplantation. The metatarsophalangeal joint (four cases), proximal interphalangeal joint (two cases), and proximal interphalangeal joint of a useless finger (one case) were used to reconstruct proximal interphalangeal and metacarpophalangeal joints in the hand or thumb. Stability, absence of pain, and continued growth occurred in six of the seven patients. Range of motion ranged from 15–50°.

The technique of second-toe transplantation is described in two patients. In one patient who had sustained an amputation of all four fingers at the metacarpophalangeal joint level, the toe was placed in the index finger position. In the other patient, whose ring finger was reconstructed after it had been amputated at the proximal interphalangeal joint, the procedure must be considered to have been primarily cosmetic.

Gait is analyzed after removal of the great toe.

This article analyzes the results in a series of great toe transplantations. Subjective assessment by the patient, objective measurements of pinch and grip, and details of the patients' work histories are given.

Reconstruction of the metacarpophalangeal and proximal interphalangeal joints of the finger and thumb is described in six patients who underwent proximal interphalangeal joint transplantation from the toes. Details of the anatomy, surgical technique, and results are presented.

This article analyzes the technical factors involved in successful toe transplantation, and should be useful to those preparing for this procedure. Anatomic variations are emphasized. Wei found the dorsalis pedis to be absent in 4% of the patients, and to have an abnormal origin in 5%.

This article describes composite joint reconstruction in toe transplantation using the joint surfaces of the proximal phalanx of the toe and the metacarpal of the thumb.

Foot-to-hand joint transplantation is described in two patients. In one, the metatarsophalangeal toe joint was used, and the proximal interphalangeal toe joint was used in the other patient. Nonvascularized joint transplantation, epiphyseal transplantation, and vascularized joint transplantation are discussed.

Wu JB, et al (1980) The distribution of arteries supplying the dorsum and planta of the foot. Acta Anat Sinica 11:13

Arterial anatomy and its variations in 100 cadaver feet are described in detail. The dorsalis pedis was absent in 4% of the feet; it originated from the fibular artery in 3%, and from the perforating branches of the tibial or fibular arteries in 2%. The first dorsal metatarsal artery arose dorsally in 51%, and from the plantar aspect in 49%. In most cases, the first dorsal metatarsal artery lay within the first interosseous muscle. It was subcutaneous in only 11%.

Zhong-Jig, Ho GH, Chen TCH (1984) Microsurgical reconstruction of the amputated hand. J Reconstr Microsurg 1:162

Sixteen cases of toe transplantation for hand reconstruction after uni- and bilateral amputation are described. One prerequisite of reconstruction was possession of a forearm at least two thirds of its original length. Artificial metacarpals were used in conjunction with the toe transplants.

5
Replantation

5.1 Indications

In the 1970s, when the possibilities for replantation were relatively unexplored, this procedure was thought to be appropriate only for clean-cut, "guillotine-type" amputations. Within 5–10 years, however, many adventurous attempts accomplished the salvage of avulsed or mangled parts. More cautious surgeons objected, citing poor ultimate function following such injuries. Uncertainty and controversy abounded, and the distinction between the kind of injuries that should be replanted and those that should be amputated was unclear. Eventually, many replantation centers generated reports of large series of patients, and these reports began to clarify the indications for replantation (Chow et al. 1979, May et al. 1982, O'Brien et al. 1974, Tamai 1982, Urbaniak et al. 1985, Weiland et al. 1977). While these indications continue to evolve and do depend partly on the experience, skill, and opinion of the surgeon, each injury can be analyzed with regard to some basic prognostic features.

One must individualize the decision of whether or not to replant a part in each case by considering **personal factors**.

Occupation and hobbies. The need for five-fingered activities such as using a keyboard or playing a musical instrument must be assessed. Some patients may require a strong tubular grasp. Also, the need to return to work as soon as possible may be a relative contraindication for replantation, which requires many months of therapy to achieve a satisfactory result.

Personal preferences. Cultural pressures may influence the priority of restoring an amputated part. Each individual views the loss of a body part differently. The longer hospital stays (7–10 days) and rehabilitation period (2–6 months) are the reasons that some patients prefer amputation closure. It should be remembered that amputation closure does not necessarily solve or end the patient's problem. Neuroma formation, skin adherence or sensitivity, poor sensation, lack of dexter-

ity, or poor pinch and grasp can all complicate single- or multiple-digit amputations.

The **patient's general condition**, both physical and mental, must be considered. When *other major injuries* contraindicate the replantation of digits, the latter assumes secondary importance. *Mental status* is always a difficult factor to assess in the emergency situation, as patients who are unstable or depressed may respond to psychiatric treatment and return to a productive life. For this reason, psychiatric factors alone should very seldom contraindicate replantation. I would proceed with replantation under most circumstances, except where chronic or permanent psychiatric illness makes cooperation with the rehabilitation program impossible. It is important to discuss these factors with the patient's mental health care professional.

The following approach to the indications for replantation relates **site and type of injury** to the likely functional outcome.

5.1.1 Single-Finger Amputations (Phelps et al. 1978, Urbaniak et al. 1985)

Single-finger replantation should be performed for the occasional patient who has strong cosmetic, psychologic, or cultural reasons for wanting the procedure done. Certain functional considerations may be important, such as if the patient is a performing musician or uses a keyboard as part of his or her occupational duties. Single-digit replantation should only be attempted with the following considerations kept in mind regarding level of injury.

5.1.1.1 Distal Phalanx

The *digital artery* trifurcates between the distal interphalangeal joint and the base of the nail. In general, arterial anastomoses are possible proximal to this trifurcation, but replantation of an amputated fingertip is difficult if it is to be performed distal to a point 2–3 mm proximal to the base of the nail. In distal am-

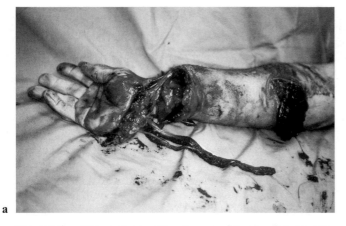

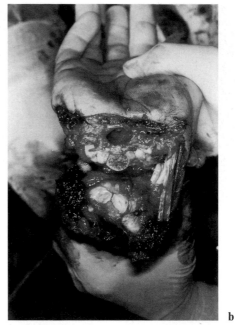

Fig. 5-14. a. This patient suffered an avulsive partial amputation at wrist level when he caught his hand in an industrial ice-crushing machine. Despite the avulsive nature of the injury, revascularization was successful. (Most amputations at this level should be replanted because of the marked disability that results from amputation of an entire hand. Also, fasciotomy of all forearm and hand compartments is essential when a crush injury is followed by ischemia.) **b.** The amputation cut through the carpus. The empty carpal tunnel is seen. Initially, the carpus was pinned; this was followed 6 months later with wrist fusion. **c** and **d.** An adequate result was achieved, with functional sensation and grasp (Fig. 2-2).

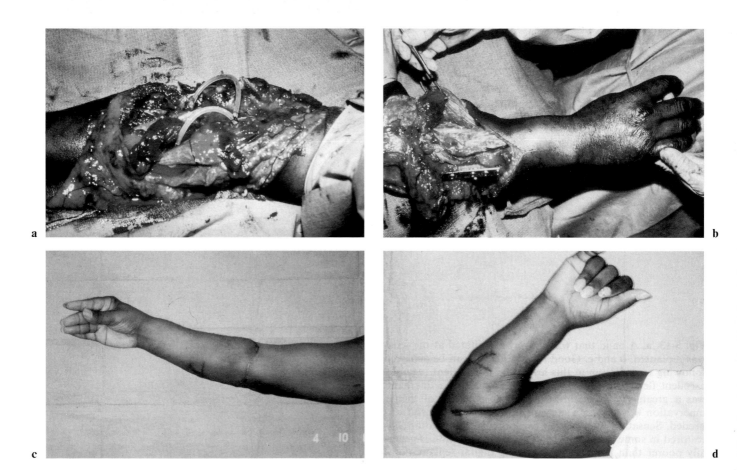

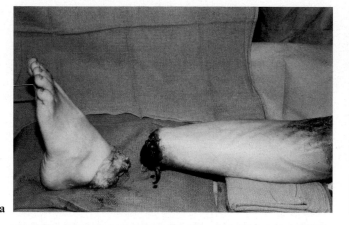

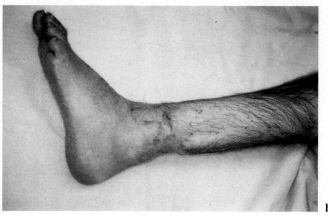

Fig. 5-16. a. This sharp amputation just proximal to the ankle required only 2 cm of shortening, and the posterior tibial nerve was in good condition on both sides of the amputation. Under these circumstances, replantation of a lower extremity is reasonable. **b.** An adequate functional result was achieved with protective sensation on the sole of the foot and a stable ankle. The patient walks with an imperceptible limp, and he has mild pain.

5.1.6 Above-Elbow Amputations (Malt and McKhan 1978, O'Brien et al. 1974)

Children fare better than adults following replantation at any level. Their regenerative potential is well known to hand surgeons, and justifies a limb salvage attempt that may not be appropriate in an older individual. Above-elbow amputations fall into this category. In adults, replantation above the elbow may be considered if there is a reasonable possibility of salvage and later function of the elbow. An attempt at salvage is justified when one considers the functional difference between an above-elbow and a below-elbow prosthesis.

In many situations, replantation above the elbow is doomed to a poor functional outcome, with the patient undergoing multiple procedures over a period of several years. Faced with that option, the patient would be far better served by closure of the amputation stump. Replantation is contraindicated in the presence of crushed or injured muscle, extensive nerve damage, or concomitant brachial plexus injury or avulsion (Fig. 5-17a).

Fig. 5-15. a. This patient suffered an amputation at the proximal forearm level in a car accident. Because the patient arrived 4 hours after the injury, vascular shunts (Sec. 5.4.1) were used to connect the proximal with the distal vessels and end the period of ischemia in the amputated part. **b.** The shunts were retained while irrigation, debridement, bone fixation, and tendon repair were done. Thereafter, vein grafts were used to repair the radial and ulnar arteries. **c** and **d.** A good functional result with good extension and flexion of the elbow and good flexion of all but the small finger was achieved. The patient desired no further reconstruction. Sensation in the fingers was protective.

5.1.7 Multiple-Level Amputations (Fig. 5-17e)

Successful replantation is improbable if longitudinal structures have been injured at multiple levels. Although vascular repair can technically salvage an extremity damaged in this way, nerve and tendon function is unlikely to be satisfactory.

5.1.8 Lower-Extremity Amputations

Because lower-extremity prostheses function excellently, the indications for replantation are far narrower than those for amputated upper extremities. Replantation of the lower extremity should only be attempted under the following circumstances: (1) in cases of clean-cut amputation, (2) where less than 3–4 cm of shortening is required, (3) in the distal third of the leg or around the ankle, and (4) if there is good-quality nerve tissue for repair (Figs. 5-16 and 5-17c and d).

5.2 Contraindications (Fig. 5-17)

1. *Severity of damage.* Replantation is not feasible after multiple-level injuries, in cases of severe upper-arm injury that involves the brachial plexus or has other serious nerve damage, or where there has been severe vessel damage (Fig. 5-17).
2. *Ischemia time.* Even though there have been anecdotal reports of digital replantation after ischemia times of 24 hours or longer, the duration of ischemia should be kept as short as possible. With amputations proximal to the ankle or wrist, 6 hours of ischemia is the upper limit for safe replantation because muscle tissue is present in the amputated part (Sec. 5.1.5).
3. *Single-digit amputations.* Replantation of digits

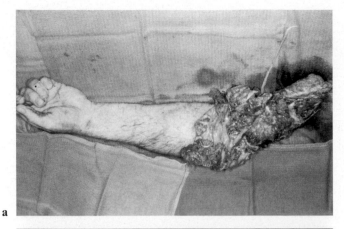

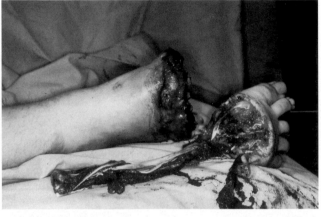

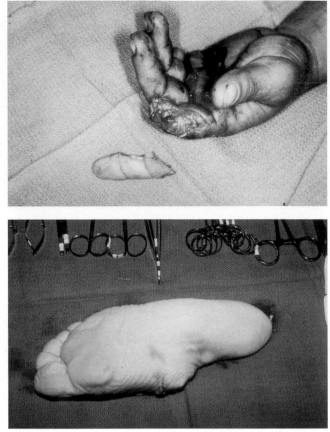

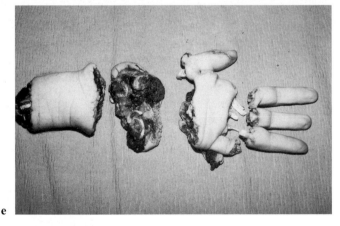

Fig. 5-17a–e. The following injuries should not be replanted: **a.** Injuries that involve avulsion of major nerves of an extremity, such as the brachial plexus. **b.** Amputations of a single finger proximal to the flexor digitorum superficialis tendon insertion, or where the proximal interphalangeal joint has been severely damaged – with poor motion at the proximal interphalangeal joint, the finger is likely to be an obstacle to good hand function (Fig. 5-2). **c.** Crush or avulsion injuries of the lower extremity – if replanted, these parts will function poorly. **d.** Injuries in which the vessels have been avulsed. The "ribbon sign" results from hemorrhage along the course of a vessel and reflects avulsive damage to it. This sign is a predictor of failure of vascular repair, and can be seen in this foot. It will also be apparent following similar injuries in fingers. **e.** Multiple-level injuries – because these require multiple arterial, nerve, and tendon repairs, the ultimate function will not be adequate.

should not be performed when the amputation is proximal to the flexor digitorum superficialis insertion, or when there is severe injury to the proximal interphalangeal joint.

In my experience, *age* has not been a contraindication to replantation (Sekiguchi and Ohmori 1979). Some motivated senior citizens have done excellently in using their replanted parts, so motivation is more important than age. Unfortunately, this factor is difficult to assess in the emergency situation.

5.3 Emergency Department Care

The UCSF Hand and Microsurgery Service suggests the following protocol for the emergency department management of patients with amputated and/or devascularized parts.

1. **Stabilize the patient**. Start a large-bore intravenous line and administer a cephalosporin intravenously. Give tetanus prophylaxis as needed. Do not give the patient anything by mouth.

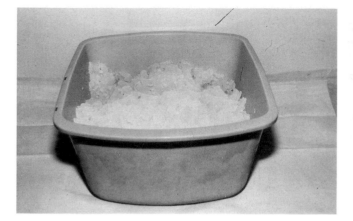

Fig. 5-18. Amputated fingers should be placed in a slightly moist sponge which is then placed in a dry, clean container. This container, in turn, is placed in a larger one containing ice. The amputated parts are not placed in direct contact with the ice, and dry ice is never used. In partial amputations, a plastic bag containing crushed ice is placed around the devascularized part. Crushed ice will conform to the contour of the amputated part better than ice cubes.

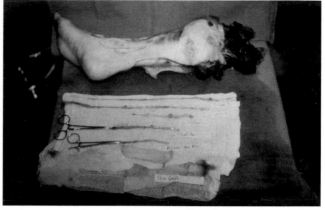

Fig. 5-19. Any amputated part that is not replantable should be used for "spare parts." This leg was not replantable, but nerve, vessel, and skin grafts were harvested to repair other injuries. Tissue transplants can also be harvested, often from donor sites that are not normally available; for example, when a foot cannot be replanted, the sole can be used as a free tissue transfer, or multiple toes can be combined with skin flaps.

2. **Prepare the amputated or devascularized part**. Cool the amputated part with regular ice as follows: If *completely amputated*, place the part in a dry container, and put this container in a larger one filled with ice (do not use dry ice) (Fig. 5-18). If *incompletely amputated*, dress the injured extremity, apply a splint, and surround it with a plastic bag containing crushed ice.
3. **Care of the injured extremity**. Wrap the wound in a bulky, soft dressing that has been soaked with an antibacterial preparation, and apply a splint.

5.4 Surgical Technique – General Considerations

5.4.1 Initial Preparation

As the patient and operating room are being prepared for surgery, additional surgeons should begin *preparing the amputated parts*. The amputated part is thoroughly irrigated and debrided, and each structure is tagged. Indeed, if multiple digits have been amputated, each one can be prepared by a different surgeon before the patient even arrives at the operating suite. Also, vein, nerve, or skin grafts can be harvested from nonreplantable parts (Fig. 5-19). In the operating room, the microscope is tested and adjusted, an appropriate mattress (e.g., an eggshell or other design appropriate for long operations) is positioned, and the room is warmed.

An axillary block *anesthetic* may be adequate for short procedures but is often inadequate for operations lasting longer than 4–6 hours. Although it has the benefit of sympathetic blockade, many patients become restless or anxious and begin to move, whereupon a general anesthetic becomes necessary. For this reason, if an operation lasting many hours is anticipated, a general anesthetic is given initially.

The patient is given intravenous *antibiotics* (a *cephalosporin*) at 6-hour intervals throughout the procedure. For extremely contaminated wounds or those involving a considerable amount of ischemic muscle tissue, *tobramycin* is added to combat any gram-negative organisms. Other antibiotics may be necessary, depending on the circumstances of the injury. Following muscle ischemia and revascularization, it is important to maintain good renal flow and urine alkalinization. Intravenous *sodium bicarbonate* is administered for this purpose. In these situations, the patient's blood potassium, electrolytes, pH, and P_{CO_2} are carefully monitored. Also, urine is tested for myoglobinuria, and a urinary catheter must be placed.

As was mentioned, the *duration of ischemia* is of critical importance when muscle tissue is involved. This crucial period can be ended by using a *Scribner shunt* to restore blood flow to the amputated or devascularized part (Figs. 5-15 and 5-20). If the duration of ischemia has been very long, the shunt can be placed when the patient reaches the emergency department, but it is more safely done immediately after the patient arrives in the operating room. The smallest size Scribner shunt adapter is sutured into the proximal and distal arteries, and the communicating tubing is connected. The adapters and tubing are tied securely into place in the vessel. Once the shunt has been placed, the surgeon must remain with the patient. Should the tubing disconnect, dangerous bleeding will result because the vessel will be unable to retract. The muscle is allowed to bleed

Kirschner wires are driven retrograde into the amputated part. The fracture is reduced and the Kirschner
wires are then driven proximally. This technique is
quite simple and quick. Fixation is only fair. The
disadvantage is unavoidable involvement of the surrounding soft tissues, which makes early mobilization difficult. In addition, it is difficult to avoid im-
mobilizing adjacent joints, especially if they are near
the amputation site.

2. *Intraosseous wiring* (Gordon and Monsanto 1987).
This technique has many advantages: the adjacent
joints are left mobile, even if the amputation is close
to the joint; good fixation is achieved in all planes;
and the wires need not be removed, thereby providing long-term fixation.

A 24- or 26-gauge wire is passed through drill holes
made proximal and distal to the fracture. The fracture is reduced and the wires are twisted tight. Several patterns of application can be used, depending
on the soft-tissue exposure and lines of force in the
particular bone. Care must be taken to provide fixation in all three planes, i.e., sagittal, coronal, and
rotatory. The most frequently used patterns of application are coronal and sagittal wiring. Several other
patterns are shown in Fig. 5-24.

Intraosseous wiring can be combined with a variety of other techniques. For example, a single or
cross Kirschner wire configuration can be combined
with coronal or sagittal intraosseous wiring. For
comminuted bones, circumferential wiring is sometimes useful as an initial step, followed by any of
the various techniques described.

3. *Tension-band wiring* (Khuri 1986). This technique
provides good fixation and resists angulation into
flexion at the fracture site. As stress into flexion is
applied at the fracture, the dorsal wire tightens and
resists this force. The disadvantage is that the
Kirschner wires often have to pass through the dorsal
extensor apparatus, and when these wires are removed, the optimal fixation provided by the technique is lost.

Two parallel and longitudinally oriented
Kirschner wires are passed across the fracture site
on the dorsal aspect of the phalanx, the metacarpal,
or the wrist. Depending on the site, a 20- to 26-gauge
wire is passed across the bone distally and brought
in figure-of-eight fashion around the Kirschner wires
as they exit the bone (Fig. 5-24e). This technique
may be used successfully for fixation at the wrist
level (Fig. 5-22) or for smaller bones in the hand.
It is particularly useful for the fusion of small joints
in the hand.

4. *Plating* (Nunley et al. 1987). The use of small plates
is effective in stabilizing transverse fractures of the
metacarpals and proximal phalanges. I also use
plates in the forearm and humerus. Plates provide
solid fixation, even for slow-healing fractures, and
simplify dressing changes and postoperative therapy.
With appropriate debridement and irrigation, the infection rate following plating is extremely low.

5. *External fixation.* This technique is reserved for situations where extensive bone loss requires later bone
grafting.

Primary silicone arthroplasty can replace a joint that
is completely destroyed if the wound is relatively clean.
However, stiffness results from periarticular swelling
and fibrosis, and seldom from incongruity of the joint
surfaces. Primary silicone arthroplasties have therefore
not been effective in providing good mobility.

5.4.6 Tendon Repairs

Flexor tenorrhaphy is performed with 3-0 or 4-0 nylon
suture. Any of the standard tendon suturing techniques
(e.g., the modified Kessler, the Kleinert, or the Bunnel
stitch) can be used. If tendons are being transferred
or if there is enough tendon length, a weave stitch
should be used because it provides the strongest repair.

In my experience with late tendon reconstruction,
I have often found the flexor digitorum superficialis
and flexor digitorum profundus to be markedly adher-
ent following replantation in "zone 2", making tenolysis difficult. In *zone 2*, therefore, I repair the flexor
digitorum profundus alone. In *regions without pulleys*,
such as the metacarpal region or the wrist, I repair
both tendons. Occasionally, transfer of the flexor digitorum superficialis tendon proximally to the flexor digitorum profundus tendon distally may be useful.

Tendons that have been *avulsed* from their musculo-
tendinous junctions do poorly because of edema and
fibrosis. Following this kind of tendon avulsion, bleeding into the forearm can occur, and monitoring for
compartment syndrome is important, especially if the
patient is receiving anticoagulants. If the *flexor pollicis
longus* has been avulsed, a tendon transfer may restore
flexion at the interphalangeal joint of the thumb. The
brachioradialis tendon is most frequently used for this
purpose. More commonly, a fusion of the interphalangeal joint of the thumb is preferable. Initially, pinning
of the interphalangeal joint suffices, and, if necessary,
a formal fusion procedure can be done at a later date.
Silicone tendon rods for later tendon grafting are not
useful in the acute replant situation because infection,
exposed wounds, and poor passive range of motion
of the joints limit the benefits of the technique.

5.4.7 Arterial Repair

It is important to anastomose a *normal vessel* proximally to a normal vessel distally. Careful scrutiny of the
intima under high-power magnification is essential.
Some surgeons place great emphasis on a strong
"*spurt*" of blood from the proximal artery. While this
strong spurt is reassuring, spasm of a quality vessel
can limit the force of this blood spurt from the proximal
vessel. Yet, if uncertainty persists, it is always best to
resect a greater amount of vessel and replace the injured
vessel with a reversed vein graft. In general, the distal
artery will be of adequate quality just distal to the *first*

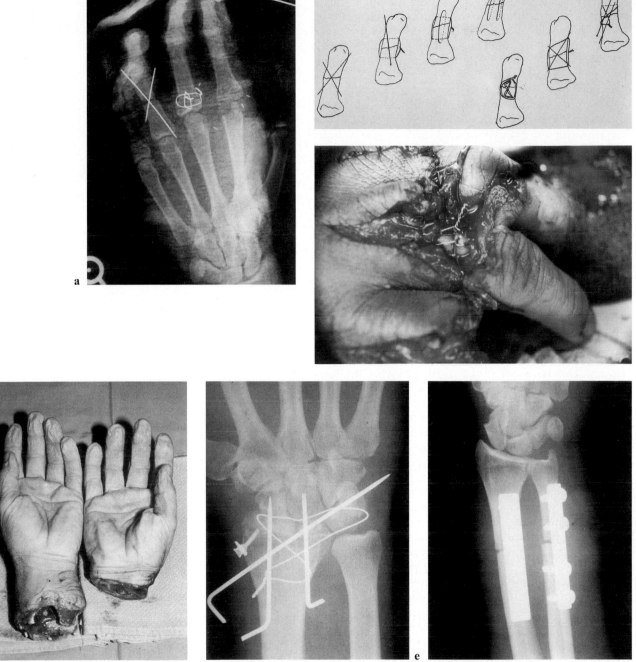

Fig. 5-24. a. Three fingers had been amputated in this patient. The ring finger was amputated at the *midportion of the proximal phalanx*, and cross Kirschner wires were used for fixation. The long finger was amputated *very close to the metacarpophalangeal joint*. In order that this joint be left free after fixation, sagittal and coronal intraosseous wiring was used to provide stabilization. The index finger was amputated *through the metacarpophalangeal joint*. A primary silicone prosthesis was placed in an attempt to retain function in this joint. (In my experience, such prostheses have not been successful in retaining good joint mobility. It is not the joint surfaces that limit motion following replantation, but *capsular and periarticular fibrosis* and *tendon adherence*, and these are not affected by silicone arthroplasty.) **b.** Any of several patterns of intraosseous wiring combined with Kirschner wiring can be used. **c.** The fractures in this amputation just distal to the metacarpophalangeal joint were fixed with two intraosseous wires which provided both angular and rotatory fixation (Fig. 5-22). **d.** This patient sustained amputations of both hands. **e.** In the amputation that occurred through the wrist, AO figure-of-eight tension band wiring was used in combination with cross Kirschner wires. **f.** In more proximal amputations, plating is the best method of fixation. Plates provide stability and do not impede mobility, rehabilitation, or dressing changes. Except for the most contaminated wounds, the infection rate following plating appears to be no greater than that occurring with other fixation techniques. Meticulous debridement and irrigation are always essential, however.

intact branch (and vice versa for the proximal vessel). When *vein grafts* are used as arterial grafts, they should be placed under mild tension because they will elongate once flow is reestablished. All small branches of the vein graft should be carefully tied with 9-0 nylon suture to prevent later spasm. Larger branches are tied with 6-0 silk to prevent bleeding when the pressure within the lumen increases with flow.

Transposition of arteries from one digit to another may simplify vascular repairs (Nakamura et al. 1980). The use of Y-shaped vein grafts is also helpful when one is fortunate enough to find such a graft at the donor site (Jones and Jupiter 1985, Pho et al. 1979).

Positioning an amputated thumb for the arterial repair is particularly difficult. The ulnar digital artery of the thumb is considerably larger than the radial, but it cannot be easily exposed from either the palmar or the dorsal surface. This problem is greatly simplified by using one of several positioning techniques. A single longitudinal Kirschner wire is placed across the interphalangeal joint and fracture, and a second oblique wire is positioned at the fracture site, ready to be passed across it. The thumb is placed in a supine position if the ulnar artery is approached from the palmar side, or pronated if this artery is approached from the dorsal side. The vein graft is anastomosed to the ulnar artery in the thumb, the thumb is rotated back into the correct position, and the second wire is driven across the fracture. Alternatively, one can suture a vein graft to this ulnar digital artery prior to replacing the thumb (Pho et al. 1979, Shafiroff and Palmer 1981).

Once resection back to the normal artery or vein has been accomplished and the vessel is irrigated with heparin (100 units/cc) prior to the anastomosis, the vessel ends are dilated gently and the repair is done. I generally repair the artery first, followed by the nerve that accompanies it, and then turn the hand over to anastomose the vein. If possible, all repairs are done under *tourniquet control*. This approach has two virtues. First, bleeding is minimal and the repairs can be done simply and quickly. Second, the hyperemic phase after the tourniquet is released may improve circulation to the replanted digit. Once the tourniquet has been released, it should not be reinflated in the face of fresh anastomoses, as stagnant blood at the site of these anastomoses can initiate thrombosis. Therefore, with multiple-digit amputations, all anastomoses but those in the initial digit are generally performed with the tourniquet deflated.

Following vascular repair, the restoration of distal circulation may be slow. The rate at which circulation is restored may depend on the duration of ischemia. Failure to restore flow in the face of patent anastomoses may result from distal capillary and cellular damage that was probably caused by prolonged ischemia. Other causes of slow return of circulation must be considered, the most common being vessel spasm.

I take the following steps when spasm is thought to be responsible for inadequate distal flow:

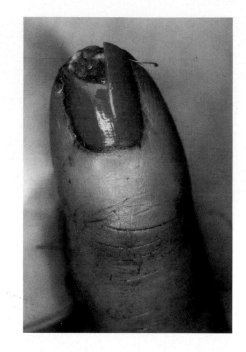

Fig. 5-25. Removal of a small part of the nail allows bleeding from the nail bed. If this area dries out, more nail can be removed.

Local Measures
1. A patency test is performed to ensure that the anastomosis is open.
2. Using a 25-gauge needle, topical bupivacaine HCl is delivered under mild pressure along the course of the vessel into the adventitia.
3. Under high-power magnification, the adventitia of the vessel is dissected and removed, and any untied small branches are ligated (even the tiniest of these can produce spasm).
4. Topical papaverine HCl is administered.
5. If available, the vessel on the opposite side of the digit is anastomosed.
6. Finally, a longer vein graft is used and the repair is redone.

Systemic Measures
1. One must make sure that a vasodilating anesthetic is being used, and one can also consider using chlorpromazine (an α-blocker) or isoxsuprine (a β-stimulant) (Sec 5.5.2). These latter two agents are more often used postoperatively.
2. Other systemic measures such as maintaining warm ambient temperature, irrigating with warm saline, and maintaining adequate blood pressure may also improve peripheral circulation and diminish vessel spasm.

5.4.8 Nerve Repairs

The nerve repair will largely dictate the functional outcome of the procedure. Nerve repairs should be done as carefully as vascular repairs, using 9-0 or 10-0 nylon suture. If mild tension is present, 8-0 suture can be

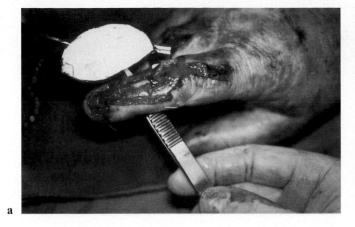

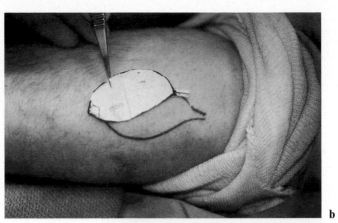

a

b

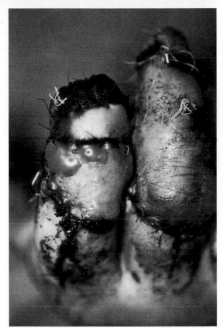

Fig. 5-26. a. This saw injury denuded the soft tissues on the dorsum of the finger. All of the fingers were badly damaged, so salvage of as much length of this index finger as possible was desirable. A vein was dissected proximally and distally, and the size of the planned flap was measured. **b.** The flap was centered over a vein in the proximal forearm. **c.** The flap is seen just proximal to a full-thickness skin graft. Despite initial congestion, the flap survived while the skin graft was lost. Enough length of the digit was salvaged for good pinch.

c

placed in the epineurium to hold the nerve together while 9-0 or 10-0 is used for subsequent stitches. I do not use primary nerve grafts because survival of the replant cannot be ensured. If the nerve is too badly damaged for repair, delayed nerve grafting 3–4 months after the replantation should be planned.

5.4.9 Venous Repairs

The dictum often quoted describes the use of two veins for each artery that has been anastomosed. If a good venous repair is accomplished with normal-looking vessels, a single vein will suffice. Indeed, it may be preferable to have a single well-repaired vein with a high rate of flow rather than multiple veins with relatively lower rates of flow. Vein grafts should be used as liberally to replace damaged segments of vein as they are to replace damaged arteries.

When performing very distal digital replantation, a vein may not be found in the amputated part, and yet venous egress must be accomplished. Several techniques can be used for this (Sec. 5.5.2).

5.4.10 Soft-Tissue Cover

Skin closure must be loose and involve as few stitches as possible. *Split-thickness skin grafts* are helpful and should be used liberally. They can successfully cover most soft tissues, including vascular grafts and anastomoses. An attempt should be made to cover tendons and fractures with full-thickness skin.

A flap containing a vein can be used to cover *dorsal or palmar finger wounds* (Yoshimura et al. 1987). Such a flap is particularly useful when a vein graft will be needed anyway. The vein graft is harvested from the proximal forearm with overlying skin, and grafted into the vein(s) of the finger (Fig. 5-26). On the *palmar surface*, skin defects can be covered with a similar flap, reversed, and anastomosed at the proximal and distal ends to a digital artery, or proximally to a digital artery and distally to a vein (Fig. 5-27). Of these combinations, the flap connected to a vein proximally and distally is the one least likely to fully survive, but it is useful if the underlying injuries preclude the use of a vein graft covered with a split-thickness skin graft.

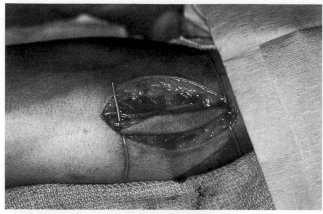
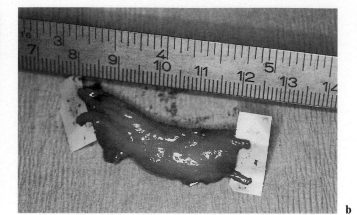
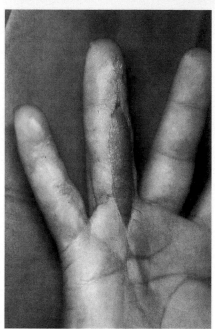

Fig. 5-27. a. This flap was centered over a forearm vein. The connections between the vein and overlying skin were carefully preserved. **b.** The deep surface of the flap is shown. **c.** The flap was reversed and interposed into the proximal and distal digital artery. The flap provided good cover over the extensive palmar digital wound.

In amputations proximal to the wrist where there has been some muscle ischemia, routine *fasciotomy* should be performed in the forearm, including both the volar and dorsal compartments (Fig. 5-28). These fasciotomy wounds should be left open and treated with skin grafting 3-4 days later or when the swelling has subsided.

5.5 Postoperative Care

Postoperatively, the patient should be in a heated room with the replanted part positioned well above the heart.

5.5.1 Dressings

Dressings should be applied extremely loosely. I use the following regimen: (1) Initially, antibiotic ointment is placed on the wounds to prevent adherence of the dressings. (2) Petrolatum gauze is then applied. Because such gauze can become caked with blood and cause constriction, it should be placed longitudinally and not circumferentially. (3) A bulky, soft dressing is then placed on both the palmar and dorsal surface, followed by a dorsal positioning splint. In the recovery room, dressings are often split down to the skin to prevent any possibility of constriction, and then loosely taped. It is important that the dressing provide warmth and allow access to the fingertips, which require monitoring.

The first dressing change can produce anxiety in the patient, which, in turn, can cause vascular spasm. If possible, the first dressing should be left in place for 4 to 5 days and then changed under adequate analgesia and sedation; this is done as a precautionary measure to avoid spasm, especially in children. A custom-made, low-temperature thermoplastic splint is then fabricated so that range-of-motion exercises can be initiated.

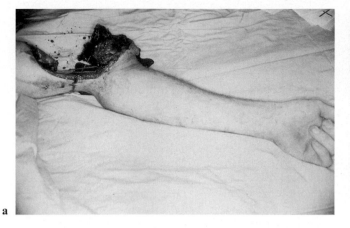

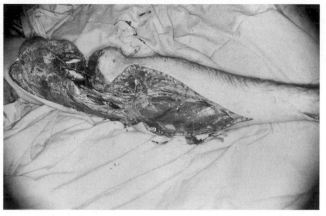

a

b

Fig. 5-28. a. This partial amputation of the upper arm was the result of a motorcycle accident. The forearm was ischemic for 4 hours afterward. **b.** The vessels were exposed and the muscle bulged as the fascia was incised. (It is extremely impor-

tant to perform a fasciotomy of all compartments in all cases where the forearm muscles have been ischemic for more than 1 hour.)

5.5.2 Postoperative Medications

Each replantation center has its own protocol regarding anticoagulants and other medications. My protocol consists of the following:

1. *Aspirin*, 325 mg daily.
2. *Dextran*. A loading dose of 50 cc intravenously is used at the beginning of the procedure. Thereafter, 30 cc/hour is given for 5–7 days.
3. *Heparin* is used in crush or avulsion injuries. After administering a loading dose of 5000 units intravenously, 1000 units/hour is given. The dose thereafter depends on the partial thromboplastin time, which is maintained at 1.5-2 times the normal value. (Heparin is never used for microvascular free tissue transplants because the large surface area of the donor site has a great potential for hematoma formation.)
4. *Chlorpromazine HCl* (5–10 mg orally every 8 hours) is used as a peripheral vasodilator only if spasm is troublesome.

In amputations at the middle or distal phalangeal level where a usable vein cannot be found, venous drainage is effected by partial nail plate removal and bleeding from the nail bed (Fig. 5-25) (Gordon et al. 1985). In this technique, a wedge of nail is removed, intravenous heparin is administered, and a heparin pledget is applied to keep the nail bed moist. This pledget is changed every 20–30 minutes. Continuous, slow bleeding from the nail bed occurs for 3–4 days. After this period, venous channels form between the replanted part and the rest of the finger, and bleeding from the nail bed diminishes. If the digit becomes congested again, more nail plate is removed. The chance of such congestion is the reason only part of the nail is removed initially.

Other techniques to accomplish venous egress, such as leeches or bleeding from the suture lines, are used by some surgeons after replantation at this level. Leeches have the disadvantage of being socially objectionable, and there are difficulties with locating a reliable source of supply. Because they come in contact with the patient's blood, questions of parasite, bacteria, or virus transmission must be raised. Nevertheless, they are a useful option if venous congestion cannot be treated by other methods.

5.5.3 Monitoring

There are many methods of confirming circulation to the fingertips. Indeed, an experienced observer is probably as good as any monitor, using the signs of capillary return, turgor, color, and temperature. The dusky, swollen appearance of a congested digit, or the empty, wrinkled pallor of arterial compromise can usually provide an accurate clinical assessment. Frequently, however, the signs are less dramatic, especially early in the sequence of vascular problems. Also, it is often difficult to have an experienced observer available on a 24-hour basis.

The *ideal monitor* should be noninvasive, continuous, quantitative, reliable, sensitive, and specific. The *pulse oxymeter* (Fig. 8-2a), which meets all of these requirements, operates by measuring the level of saturated hemoglobin. A drop in pressure below 90 mm Hg indicates arterial occlusion. With venous occlusion, a further drop will occur approximately 1 hour after the problem arises. This apparatus is available in most anesthesia and cardiac care departments.

If a pulse oxymeter is unavailable, the *dermal quantitative fluorimeter* can substitute, but it has two disadvantages. First, the reading is taken every 2 hours and is therefore not continuous. Second, it requires a 1-cc intravenous injection of fluorescein, which occasionally produces nausea or an allergic reaction. With this method, a baseline reading is taken. Fluorescein is then injected intravenously (1 cc for an average-size adult). A second reading is taken 10 minutes later. A rise of at least 30% will occur if arterial circulation is intact. A reading taken 1 hour after injection will show a slow runoff with a decrease in the fluorescein value. If this decrease does not occur, the diagnosis of venous congestion can be made (Graham et al. 1985). This cycle is repeated every 2 hours, which is the renal clearance time of fluorescein.

5.5.4 Reexploration (Biemer 1981, Moneim and Chacon 1985)

When there is evidence of arterial or venous thrombosis, the part should be reexplored immediately. Patients are given nothing by mouth for 24 hours after surgery because of the possibility that reexploration may be necessary. If arterial or venous thrombosis is diagnosed early enough (within 1–2 hours), the other vessel (artery or vein) may still have flow. Heparin is useful in preventing thrombosis in these vessels. While many medications such as heparin and streptokinase have been advocated for the treatment of thrombosis, they are rarely indicated or effective when used alone. Reexploration is the only method that will provide reliable salvage. A salvage rate of 60–70% can usually be achieved with the use of vein grafts if the vascular problem is detected early enough.

5.5.5 Hand Therapy and Rehabilitation Program
– by Pam Silverman, O.T.R.

The hand therapist becomes involved in the rehabilitation program within the second or third day after surgery. The therapist and surgeon review the structures that have been repaired, the level of the fractures, the nature of the injury, and then discuss any precautions that must be observed in the initial management. The first dressing is generally changed about 4–5 days after surgery. This dressing change should be done sooner if there has been excessive bleeding or if there is any question that the dressing is constrictive. In cases where the amputation was proximal to the wrist and there is a large amount of muscle tissue in the replanted part, dressings should be changed daily because swelling and muscle necrosis predispose the patient to infection and subsequent vascular problems. Regular dressing changes allow an early diagnosis of such problems.

0 to 10 Days (Acute Phase)

Once it is removed, the bulky, soft dressing is replaced and the therapist carefully designs and fabricates a static dorsal positioning splint. In the initial evaluation and treatment planning, the therapist must take into ac-count the stability and level of the fracture, the level of the amputation, the level of the vascular and neural repairs, the location of tendon repair, and the type and condition of skin closure and any grafting. The wrist is positioned in neutral for more proximal amputations, and in slight flexion for amputations at or distal to the midpalmar crease. The metacarpophalangeal joints are held in gentle flexion and the interphalangeal joints are extended. The digits are secured with a wide and soft strap. Once the wounds are stable, the therapist can begin daily dressing changes with the help of the nursing staff.

In digital replantation, early protective motion (EPM I) is initiated on the fifth postoperative day. EPM I consists of simple tenodesis exercises, with gentle wrist flexion. This position allows the metacarpophalangeal joints and interphalangeal joints to gently extend. The wrist is then brought to a neutral position with simultaneous flexion at the metacarpophalangeal and interphalangeal joints.

10 Days to 3 Weeks

At this point, the next stage of early protective motion (EPM II) is begun. EPM II involves the following: (1) The wrist is positioned in *neutral* and the fingers are brought into an *intrinsic-plus* position, with the metacarpophalangeal joints flexed and the interphalangeal joints extended. The patient is asked to *hold* this position. (2) From the above *intrinsic-plus* position, the digits are carefully placed in a *claw* or *intrinsic-minus* position, with the metacarpophalangeal joints in extension and the proximal interphalangeal and distal interphalangeal joints gently flexed. The patient again holds this position. Edema and pin placement may initially limit these positions.

Certain precautions must be taken:

1. Proximal interphalangeal joint flexion should be limited to 60° if there is a zone 2 extensor tendon repair. The extensor tendons generally function poorly following replantation in this region, and there is often an excessive pull of the flexor tendons, causing a late flexion contracture of both the proximal interphalangeal and distal interphalangeal joints. Tenolysis of the extensor tendons is difficult and often unrewarding. For this reason, the extensor tendons should be favored and flexion of the fingers limited.
2. If there is a nerve or vascular repair at the proximal interphalangeal joint level, motion should be limited to approximately 30° of extension until about 3 weeks, at which time it is safe to proceed without risk of damage.
3. The claw position is begun as a passive exercise. It progresses to an active exercise at approximately 10–14 days.
4. If the level of tendon repair is distal to the proximal interphalangeal joint and the flexor tendon has been repaired, the dorsal blocking splint should be com-

bined with a palmar platform splint; this discourages development of a mallet finger, and flexion/extension should be limited to approximately 10° at the distal interphalangeal joint. In zone 2 injuries, more distal interphalangeal joint motion is permissible, but only if the finger is maintained in extension between hand therapy sessions.

3 to 8 Weeks

The range-of-motion exercises are continued, with passive and active composite motion permitted at approximately 4 weeks. In addition, dynamic splinting with rubber bands is also instituted at about 4 weeks, with alternating composite extension and flexion. These splints are frequently needed following digital replantation to increase composite passive motion. Muscle reeducation, activities that promote dexterity, and progressive resistive exercises are begun at about 8 weeks.

Other aspects of hand function receive attention, depending on the particular needs of the patient. *Edema control* with retrograde massage, compressive wrapping, and contrast baths are begun at approximately 3 to 4 weeks. Vascular supply and pain must be monitored. The edema control techniques may also decrease pain. If *desensitization* is necessary, vibration techniques and dowels are useful. Compression gloves can be prescribed after 8 weeks.

As wound care, motion, and attention to hand function continue, many other facets of the patient's rehabilitation program must be considered. The patient's reaction to injury and motivation are perhaps the most important factors in the rehabilitation process. *Psycho-*

logic supportive measures are extremely important. Early reintegration of the individual back into the workplace is particularly helpful in this regard, especially if the employer can provide a light-duty position. Anything that brings the patient closer to functioning as he or she did prior to the injury is beneficial. Work hardening programs, job retraining, and dominance change must all be considered at the appropriate time.

Any *reconstructive surgery* is generally undertaken once hand swelling and inflammation have resolved. This resolution generally takes about 6 months. Finally, the "team approach" in handling these complex injuries can markedly improve the result. It is therefore important to include family and other support systems as well as insurance companies, rehabilitation nurses, and vocational counselors in the rehabilitation program.

5.5.6 Late Reconstruction (Figs. 5-29 and 5-30)

To restore the best possible function, later reconstruction is often necessary. It is important to wait for all inflammation and swelling to subside before proceeding; this usually takes about 6 months, but it may be longer if foreign material is present, if there has been infection, or in cases of crush injury. The most common reconstructive procedures are tenolysis, tendon reconstruction, and nerve grafting (Fig. 5-29). If tenolysis is not possible and tendon grafting is necessary, two-stage reconstruction is almost always needed because of the magnitude of these injuries and their propensity for scarring (Fig. 5-30).

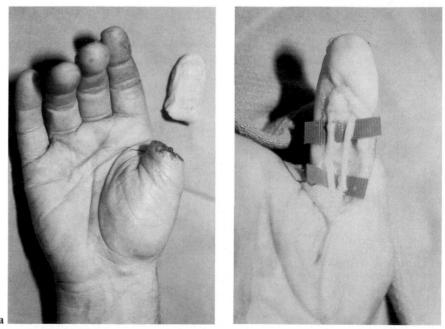

Fig. 5-29. a. This sharply amputated thumb was replanted. **b.** Two nerve grafts were performed to improve sensation. **c** and **d.** Good mobility and 8-mm two-point discrimination were achieved (see next page).

a   b

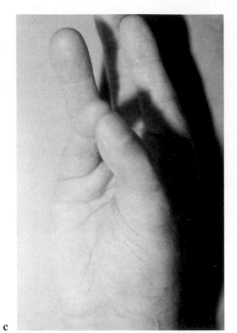

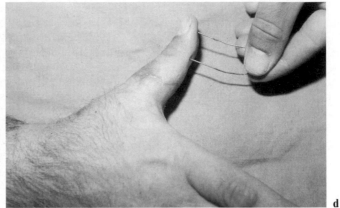

Fig. 5-29 c, d

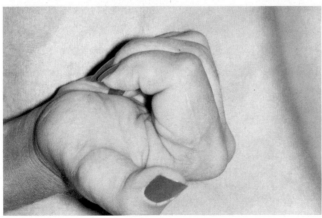

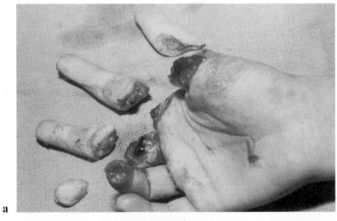

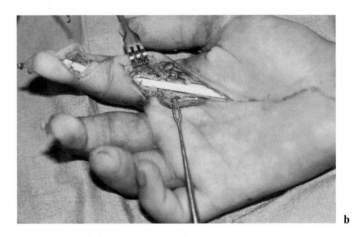

Fig. 5-30. a. This patient's thumb and three fingers were amputated by a tile-making machine. b. Poor flexor tendon excursion required tendon reconstruction. (A two-staged reconstruction using silicone rods is almost always needed following these injuries.) c. A good functional result was achieved.

5.6 Surgical Technique

5.6.1 Thumb Replantation (Fig. 5-31)

a. This 35-year-old patient was involved in a roping accident and sustained an amputation of the thumb at the interphalangeal joint level. Because this was an avulsive injury, vein grafts were planned.

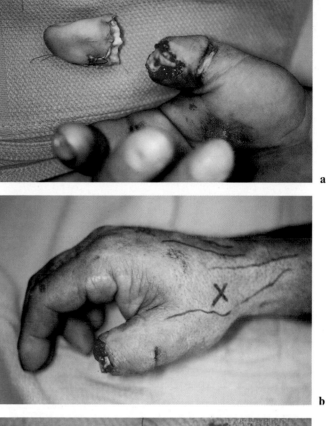

b. The radial artery is palpated and marked on the dorsal aspect of the hand between the first and second metacarpals. The veins are outlined; these are planned as the recipient vessels.

c. The amputated part is prepared by tagging the *digital artery and nerve* on both sides and dissecting a dorsal vein.

d. A vein graft is harvested from the foot and taken to another table where it is sutured to the *ulnar digital artery* and a dorsal vein. In the thumb, the ulnar digital artery is always much larger than the radial artery.

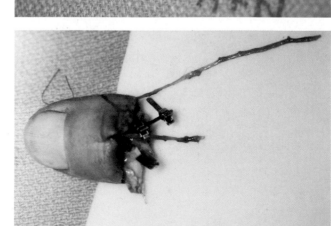

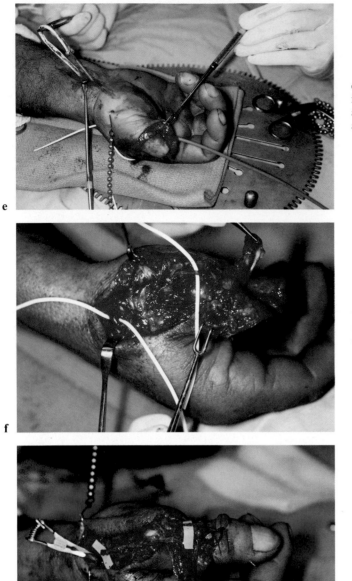

e. The *extensor pollicis longus* and *flexor pollicis longus* are identified. The flexor pollicis longus is sutured to a catheter and delivered into the distal wound. The digital nerves are also dissected and tagged on the palmar surface.

f. Three structures are dissected and tagged on the dorsal surface: (1) the radial artery, (2) a dorsal vein, and (3) the extensor tendon.

g. Thumb fixation is performed with cross Kirschner wires passed retrograde into the amputated part, which is then positioned on the amputation stump. The Kirschner wires are then passed proximally into the proximal phalanx. Next, the dorsal vein is repaired. The vein graft connecting the ulnar digital artery to the radial artery is then anastomosed end-to-side to the radial artery. The skin is closed loosely.

5.6.2 Digital Replantation
(Fig. 5-32; see also Fig. 5-21)

a. A 45-year-old man sustained a saw injury to all of the fingers of his right hand. After inspecting the amputated part, it is evident that the artery of the amputated small finger is injured too distally for replantation, but the proximal interphalangeal joint in this finger is intact on the hand. The index finger is too badly damaged to salvage. The overall situation makes digital transposition advisable in order to salvage as many fingers with intact proximal interphalangeal joints as possible.

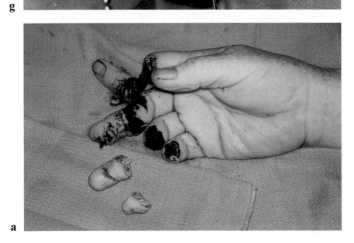

b. The index finger is inspected and the distal part is found to have an adequate neurovascular bundle, but the damage proximally precludes its replantation.

c. The amputated index finger is dissected through an incision just dorsal to the neurovascular bundle. The nerve can be seen with the artery just dorsal to it.

d. The dorsal skin flap is then raised off the extensor tendon, and, on inspection of the deep surface of this flap, veins can be identified. A vein has been dissected and tagged.

e. The neurovascular bundles are identified in the amputation stumps. The artery and nerve are dissected through incisions just posterior to the midaxial line. The arteries and nerves are tagged with 6-0 silk suture. The flexor and extensor tendons are also identified. An incision at the midpalmar crease may be necessary to identify the flexor tendon and deliver it into the distal wound. These tendons are then tagged with 3-0 nylon.

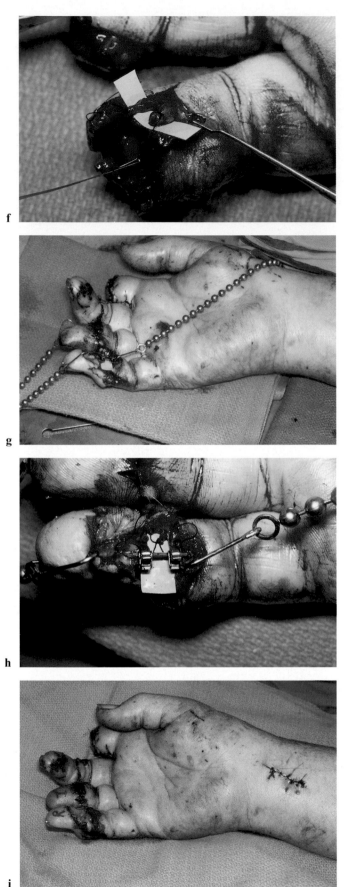

f. A close-up of these structures.

g. Appropriate retraction is important and the fingers are positioned so that exposure is not impeded.

h. The bone fixation is accomplished (Sec. 5.4.5) (Fig. 5-24) and the flexor tendon is then repaired. Repair of one or both digital arteries and both digital nerves is performed.

i. At the end of the procedure, there are three fingers with good neurovascular repair and intact proximal interphalangeal joints. The index finger is in the ring finger position, and the ring finger is in the small finger position (Fig. 5-21).

5.6.3 Ring Avulsion Injury (Fig. 5-33)

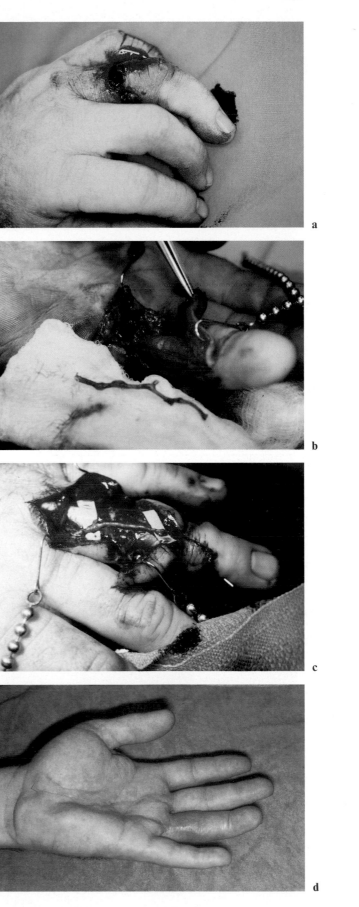

a. This 38-year-old fireman sustained a ring avulsion injury with devascularization of the finger and avulsion of the soft tissues to the distal phalangeal level.

b. Both digital nerves are intact, but the digital arteries have been severely damaged and the digit has no vascularity. A vein graft has been harvested and reversed for use in the arterial reconstruction. The artery must be resected proximally and distally back to where it is normal. After transecting the artery, the intima should appear normal under high-power magnification. Often, the first normal segment of artery will be beyond the first uninjured branch.

c. A vein graft is also used to repair the vein.

d and e. An excellent functional result with normal sensation can be achieved following this type of injury.

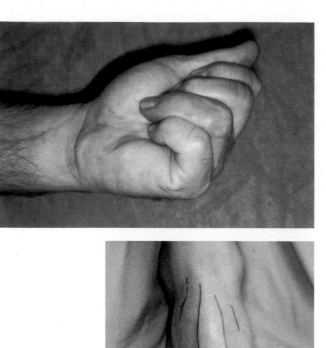

Fig. 5.33e

5.6.4 Vein Graft Harvesting (Fig. 5-34)

a. The thigh tourniquet is adjusted so that blood pressure is between systolic and diastolic; this makes the veins on the dorsal aspect of the foot and ankle stand out so that they can be marked. The smaller of the veins on the dorsum of the foot are generally of appropriate size for use in the fingers. The veins found at the ankle are used for wrist and more proximal repairs.

b. In dissecting the veins, all side branches are tied. The small branches are tied on the side closest to the parent vein with 9-0 nylon suture while the larger ones are tied with 6-0 silk. The opposite side can be coagulated with a bipolar coagulator. Heparinized saline (100 units/cc) is flushed through the vein graft prior to its use. One end of the vein graft is marked to make sure the vein will be appropriately reversed for arterial repairs; otherwise, venous valves will not allow blood flow. Great care in vein harvesting will decrease the problems of spasm and leakage at the recipient site.

5.7 Selected Bibliography

Biemer E (1981) Salvage operations for complications following replantation and free tissue transfer. Int Surg 66:37

The author found thrombosis following replantation to be largely on the venous side. He treated this with thrombectomy, heparin, dextran, and aspirin. Clinical presentation and causes are discussed. (In my experience, thrombosis occurs about as frequently in the arteries as it does in the veins. Prompt reoperation and placement of vein grafts provides the best chance of salvage.)

Chow JA, Bilos ZJ (1983) Forearm replantation. Long-term functional results. Ann Plast Surg 10:15

The surgical technique and results of forearm replantation are described. The importance of excellent nerve repair is emphasized and the authors' rehabilitation program is discussed.

Chow JA, Bilos ZJ, Chunprapaph B (1979) Thirty thumb replantations. Indications and results. Plast Reconstr Surg 64:626

Thumb function has been assessed to be 40% of hand function, so almost all thumb amputations should be replanted. The functional result is generally good. The demands for motion in the thumb are not as great as for the fingers, so most of the patients who had interphalangeal joint fusions had good thumb function. Bone was generally shortened 6–10 mm. (I feel that bone shortening should be minimized but may be indicated to allow nerve repair. For vessel damage, vein grafts are preferable to bone shortening. Shortening bone more than 10 mm should be done only rarely.)

Cooney WP III (1978) Revascularization and replantation after upper extremity trauma. Experience with interposition artery and vein grafts. Clin Orthop 137:227

The problem of failed replantation in cases of severe crush or avulsion injury is described. For improved survival, the use of patient selection criteria, interpositional artery or vein grafts for diffuse vessel damage, and anticoagulants are discussed. Some contraindications to replantation are also given.

Earley MJ (1986) The arterial supply of the thumb, first web and index finger and its surgical application. J Hand Surg 11 B:163

This article details the vasculature of the thumb, index finger, and palm, including the anomalies. Variations of the princeps pollicis artery should be noted as well as the relative vessel size that can be expected (e.g., the radial digital artery of the thumb is consistently smaller than the ulnar digital artery).

Gordon L, Leitner DW, Buncke HJ, et al (1985) Partial nail plate removal after digital replantation as an alternative method of venous drainage. J Hand Surg 10 A:360

The technique of venous outflow through the nail bed in combination with systemic anticoagulation is described. The authors consider this the method of choice for treating the problem of venous engorgement after digital replantation when venous anastomosis is not possible.

Gordon L, Monsanto EH (1987) Skeletal stabilization for digital replantation surgery. Use of intraosseous wiring. Clin Orthop 214:72

Different patterns of intraosseous wiring are described. These patterns allow mobility in the proximal and distal joints, which is important for postoperative therapy.

Graham BH, Gordon L, Alpert BS, et al (1985) Serial quantitative skin surface fluorescence. A new method for postoperative monitoring of vascular perfusion in revascularized digits. J Hand Surg 10 A:226

This method of monitoring replanted and revascularized parts is described.

Harris GD, Finseth F, Buncke HJ (1980) The hazard of cigarette smoking following digital replantation. J Microsurg 1:403

The harmful effect of cigarette smoking following replantation surgery is well known, and patients should be cautioned about this danger before their procedure.

Ikuta Y (1978) Method of bone fixation in reattachment of amputations in the upper extremities. Clin Orthop 133:169

This article discusses the surgical procedures for replanting amputated limbs and digits. The details of bone fixation of the upper arm, elbow joint, forearm, wrist joint, hand, and digits are included.

Jones NF, Jupiter JB (1985) The use of Y-shaped interposition vein grafts in multiple digit replantations. J Hand Surg 10 A:675

The use of Y-shaped vein grafts is described. The single proximal limb is anastomosed to the common digital vessels, and the two distal limbs are anastomosed to two digital arteries.

Jupiter JB (1986) Replantation. In Watson N, Smith RJ (eds): Methods and Concepts in Hand Surgery. London, Butterworths, p 270

The author describes the indications for and techniques of replantation that are used at the Massachusetts General Hospital. Some useful osteosynthesis techniques are also described.

Khuri SM (1986) Tension band arthrodesis in the hand. J Hand Surg 11 A : 41

The technique of tension band wiring for arthrodesis of small joints is described. A similar technique is used for fracture fixation.

Komatsu S, Tamai S (1968) Successful replantation of a completely cut-off thumb. Case report. Plast Reconstr Surg 42:374

This was the first report of a successful digital replant. The replanted thumb does not flex at the interphalangeal joint because the flexor tendon was not repaired. Repair of the digital nerve was postponed for fear of damaging the artery. The historic moment when circulation returned is recounted in this landmark article. (Even for today's most experienced replant surgeons, the moment when circulation returns is always accompanied by a sense of relief and accomplishment. Today, if possible, all structures are repaired at the initial replant procedure.)

Kutz JE, Hanel D, Scheker L, et al (1983) Upper extremity replantation. Orthop Clin North Am 14:873

The types of injuries encountered in replantation cases and indications for replantation are described. Cooling technique, the details and order of repair of various structures, and pitfalls (especially unrecognized blood loss) are discussed. Postoperative management is described, including some monitoring techniques.

Leung PC (1980) An analysis of complications in digital replantations. Hand 12:25

The etiology of and possible remedies for the complications of replantation are considered. Both of the early problems of vascular compromise – bleeding and infection – and the late problems of stiffness, deformity, and nonunion are discussed.

Malt RA, McKhan CF (1978) Replantation of severed arms. Clin Orthop 133:3

This is the classic and historic first case of limb replantation. The patient, a 12-year-old boy, arrived at the Massachusetts General Hospital 30 minutes after his right arm was severed below the elbow. An excellent long-term functional result was achieved, which is unusual for a replanted limb avulsed at this level, even for today. Young age and low ischemia time figure prominently in the decision to replant the entire upper limb.

May JW, Toth BA, Gardner M (1982) Digital replantation distal to the proximal interphalangeal joint. J Hand Surg 7:161

In this series of 24 replanted digits, the authors achieved a 96% survival rate and a mean active range of motion of the proximal interphalangeal joint of 95° with 11-mm two-point discrimination. Early return to school or work was possible. This group of patients who underwent replantation at this level was the first such series to be analyzed, and it is important to be familiar with this article when considering the indications for replantation.

Meyer VE (1985) Hand amputations proximal but close to the wrist joint. Prime candidates for reattachment (long-term functional results). J Hand Surg 10 A:989

This retrospective analysis of 49 hand amputations demonstrates that a generally favorable outcome can be achieved with reattachment – 80% had excellent or good results.

Moneim MS, Chacon NE (1985) Salvage of replanted parts of the upper extremity. J Bone Joint Surg 67 A:880

Fifteen replanted parts were reexplored to attempt salvage after vascular problems developed. Arterial occlusion was found in 11, while both arterial and venous occlusion occurred in four. Eight of ten vein grafts were successful. Thrombectomy was performed in six parts but was successful in only one.

Nakamura J, Kinoshita Y, Hama H, et al (1980) Successful replantation of four fingers by a single common digital artery anastomosis. J Microsurg 2:53

This article describes a case of four-finger replantation at the metacarpophalangeal joint level. All four digits survived, based on the third common palmar digital artery alone. Angiography showed transverse branches between the digital arteries on either side of the index, long, and ring fingers just proximal to the metacarpophalangeal joints. In replantations at this level (metacarpophalangeal), it may be possible to supply more than one digit through the repair of a single artery.

Nissenbaum M (1980) A surgical approach for replantation of complete digital amputations. J Hand Surg 5:58

An incision dorsal to the midaxial line allows dissection of the palmar and dorsal flaps in order to expose the digital arteries and veins. The details of exposure are described.

Nunley JA, Goldner RD, Urbaniak JR (1987) Skeletal fixation in digital replantation. Use of the "H" plate. Clin Orthop 214:66

Use of the AO H-plate is advocated for transverse fractures of the metacarpals and proximal phalanges.

Nunley JA, Koman LA, Urbaniak JR (1982) Major upper extremity replantation. Orthop Trans 6:512

Twelve complete and 27 incomplete amputations proximal to the wrist are reviewed.

Nunley JA, Spiegl PV, Goldner RD, et al (1987) Longitudinal epiphyseal growth after replantation and transplantation in children. J Hand Surg 12A:274

Epiphyseal growth continues after replantation and transplantation if the vascular supply is maintained. The average increase in length achieved during the follow-up period, which ranged from 27–81 months, was 92% of normal.

O'Brien BMcC, Macleod AM, Hayhurst JW, et al (1974) Major replantation surgery in the upper limb. Hand 6:217

Seven cases of replantation proximal to the wrist are described in detail. Three were later amputated, one for infection and two for extensive muscle and skin damage. Although the other four patients regained a functional extremity, the risks of such replantation must be kept in mind.

Phelps DB (1978) Should a torn-off little finger ever be replanted? Plast Reconstr Surg 61:592

Phelps comments on a previous article describing the replantation of a small finger that had been avulsively amputated at the metacarpophalangeal joint level. Function is unlikely to be good, but the technical possibility of replanting an avulsively amputated small finger can be extrapolated to the thumb or a multiple digit injury, in which case the indication would be different. Vein grafts should be used more or less routinely for such replantation.

Pho RWH, Chacha PB, Yeo KQ (1979) Rerouting vessels and nerves from other digits in replanting an avulsed and degloved thumb. Plast Reconstr Surg 64:330

The transfer of vessels from one digit to another is described as an alternative to vein grafting in replanting the avulsed thumb. Transfer of the dorsal digital nerves is also described.

Sekiguchi J, Ohmori K (1979) Youngest replantation with microsurgical anastomoses. Hand 11:64

Children tend to achieve excellent function following digital replantation. Replantation in children often depends on vessel size, which fortunately is often proportionally larger than expected if judging from the size of the child. Vascular spasm is often a problem, and the importance of adequate analgesia, antispasmodics, and a warm ambient temperature is emphasized. This article describes digital replantation in a 12-month-old patient.

Shafiroff BB, Palmer AK (1981) Simplified technique for replantation of the thumb. J Hand Surg 6:623

Anastomosing vein grafts to the digital vessels of an amputated thumb simplifies positioning of the hand for the vascular repairs.

Tamai S (1982) Twenty years' experience of limb replantation. Review of 293 upper extremity replants. J Hand Surg 7:549

The author discusses his extensive experience in replantation, and includes indications, levels of amputation, ischemia time, postoperative management, results, and many other factors that are important to the replant surgeon.

Tupper JW (1978) Techniques of bone fixation and clinical experience in replanted extremities. Clin Orthop 133:165

This article describes various methods of bone fixation as the first step in replantation. Vein grafting is preferred to bone shortening for direct vessel opposition. Clinical experiences with failed replants are discussed and recommendations to improve results are given.

Urbaniak JR, Evans JP, Bright DS (1981) Microvascular management of ring avulsion injuries. J Hand Surg 6:25

Ring avulsion injuries are classified and their management is described. The categories of injury are (1) *circulation adequate* – standard bone and soft-tissue treatment is adequate; (2) *circulation inadequate* – vascular reconstruction preserves viability (reasonable functional results were achieved); and (3) *complete degloving or amputation* – replantation is possible but the functional result is unpredictable. Good judgment is needed in deciding whether or not these kinds of amputations should be replanted. Results, sensation, and range of motion are reviewed.

Urbaniak JR, Hayes MG, Bright DS (1978) Management of bone in digital replantation. Free vascularized and composite bone grafts. Clin Orthop 133:184

The surgical technique of bone shortening; the management of joint injuries; and nerve, vessel, and tendon repair are described. A simple, longitudinal Kirschner wire is used for fixation. Today, more rigid fixation that does not involve the proximal or distal joints is preferred.

Urbaniak JR, Roth JH, Nunley JA, et al (1985) The results of replantation after amputation of a single finger. J Bone Joint Surg 67A:611

Fifty-nine patients who underwent single-finger replantation were reviewed; 86% of the digits survived. If the replantation was distal to the proximal interphalangeal joint, the average range of motion in that joint was 82°; if proximal to this joint, the average range of motion was 35°.

Vlaston C, Earle AS (1986) Avulsion injuries of the thumb. J Hand Surg 11A:51

Seven patients who had avulsion injuries of the thumb underwent replantation. Similarities among the injuries and the routine use of vein grafts are emphasized.

Weiland AJ, Villareal-Rios A, Kleinert HE, et al (1977) Replantation of digits and hands. Analysis of surgical techniques and results in 71 patients with 86 replantations. J Hand Surg 2:1

This article reviews 86 replants with regard to functional outcome. The patient population is described, and the location and type of injury are given. The surgical technique is detailed, and results over the 5-year period between 1970 and 1975 are reviewed. The discussion includes selection criteria and contraindications to replantation.

Yamano Y (1985) Replantation of the amputated distal part of the fingers. J Hand Surg 10A:211

The zones of replantation distal to the proximal interphalangeal joint, based on vascular anatomy, are described. Arteries in zone 1 (just proximal to the nail) were anastomosed, and venous egress was provided by "fishmouth drip vessels." Other authors have used leeches (Foucher G [1986] J Hand Surg 11A:456) or bleeding through the nail bed (Gordon et al. 1985) to accomplish venous egress. Experience with 87 digits is described.

Yoshimura M, Shimada T, Imura S, et al (1987) The venous skin graft method for repairing skin defects of the fingers. Plast Reconstr Surg 79:243

The technique and use of small flaps nourished by an underlying vein are described.

Regional Indications

6.1 Soft Tissue

The potential benefits of microvascular tissue transplantation are outlined in Sec. 2.1. Free tissue transplantation enables immediate elevation of the injured part, early mobilization in hand cases, and reconstruction in a single operation. As important as all of these factors is the advantage of being able to choose from a variety of different tissues. This allows the surgeon to tailor the surgical solution to the specific nature, site, and size of the clinical problem. A tissue that satisfies a number of requirements can be chosen. The various attributes to be found among the different tissues include variable size, vascularity, the ability to contour to the wound's dead space, sensation, limited mobility of the flap on the deeper tissues, and the ability to be combined with bone to form a composite transplant for the treatment of combined soft-tissue and bone defects. Once the decision to perform a microvascular transplant has been made, the choice of tissue must be carefully considered.

6.1.1 The Hand

6.1.1.1 Dorsum

If the tendons and paratenon are intact, split-thickness skin grafting generally suffices. If they are not intact, if bone is exposed or missing, or if later tendon reconstruction will be needed, a microvascular transplant may be the best solution. Thin, pliable skin with a mobile subcutaneous layer is needed to mimic the skin that naturally occurs in this region, and to allow subsequent tendon reconstruction. The *lateral arm flap* (Fig. 2-5) is ideal for this purpose. The *scapular flap* (Figs. 2-2 and 2-4) is more bulky but can be used for large defects that involve the forearm. The *dorsalis pedis flap* (Fig. 2-1) is of appropriate thickness, but the donor site is a problem and outweighs the primary advantage

of this flap in providing sensation. Muscle or fascial flaps are not as pliable, and tendon reconstruction is more difficult under these flaps compared with cutaneous flaps. Two-stage tendon reconstruction is used routinely under muscle flaps.

If both the dorsum and palm need cover, separate slips of the *serratus anterior* can be applied to both sides of the hand (Fig. 1-5). Massive injuries may require a very large flap to drape over the hand, in which case the *latissimus dorsi* transplant can be used (Fig. 1-8). Occasionally, a composite transplant which consists of bone and soft tissue will be needed. The *composite dorsalis pedis transplant*, which includes the second metatarsal or metatarsophalangeal joint and tendons, can be used for a single metacarpal (Figs. 4-19 and 4-24). The *iliac crest osteocutaneous* transplant can be used for multiple metacarpal loss that occurs in conjunction with an extensive soft-tissue wound.

6.1.1.2 Palm

While cutaneous flaps are often too mobile to be ideal cover in the palm, the *serratus anterior muscle flap* is small and contours well (Figs. 1-4, 1-6, and 1-7). The split-thickness skin graft tends to be quite serviceable, and breakdown is unusual. Another option is the *lateral arm flap*, and for small defects, a narrow *dorsalis pedis flap* is useful (Fig. 2-1). Both the dorsalis pedis and lateral arm flaps provide sensation, which is an advantage when they are used in the palm. These flaps can be tailored to treat defects on adjacent fingers (Fig. 2-9). The *"retrograde" radial forearm flap*, also an option for the palm, is thin and can regain sensation (Fig. 2-7).

6.1.2 Upper Arm

The latissimus dorsi can be mobilized with or without a cutaneous component and be brought subcutaneously down the upper arm to cover most defects in the upper arm or elbow region. Dissection of the neurovascular pedicle and division of the muscle insertion allows more distant transfer of the muscle. If the latissimus dorsi and other local flaps are unavailable, microvascular transplantation may be necessary.

6.1.3 Forearm

Frequently, *groin or abdominal pedicle flaps* can be used in this region. If infection is present, a *microvascular muscle flap* may be preferable (Fig. 1-3). Major acute wounds may also be treated with a *microvascular cutaneous flap*, which allows elevation of the extremity and early hand therapy (Fig. 2-2). Because muscle flaps may break down if used across major flexion creases, a musculocutaneous transplant is often preferable, placing the cutaneous portion of the transplant across the flexion crease (Fig. 1-26).

6.1.4 Heel

Reconstruction of the heel remains an extremely difficult challenge. Subsequent breakdown, pain, and difficulties with ambulation are all evidence of the repeated pressure between the ground and the calcaneus. Following a devascularizing injury of the heel, it is difficult to ascertain how much tissue will become necrotic (Figs. 1-19 and 1-21). Because of the skin's thickness in this region, it takes 7–10 days before the amount of necrosis becomes evident.

Ideally, the tissue replacement should have limited *shear* on the deeper structures, some sensation, and be a good match in terms of size. Muscle tissue has little mobility early on, but it tends to become more mobile as it atrophies, and several debulking procedures are usually necessary. Still, muscle tissue or fascia is better than a purely cutaneous flap.

The *dorsalis pedis flap*, *lateral arm flap* (Figs. 2-3 and 2-6), *deltoid flap*, and *tensor fasciae latae transplant* (Fig. 1-21) all have the potential for *sensory return*. The choice among these flaps depends on the defect size (Fig. 1-1). The tensor fasciae latae flap must be oriented longitudinally along the sole. If placed transversely, it will be too bulky. If none of these flaps will be of appropriate size, the latissimus dorsi musculocutaneous transplant may be useful in some situations (Fig. 1-19).

6.1.5 Leg and Thigh

For a variety of clinical problems in the leg, microvascular transplants should be used when rotation flaps or other local procedures will be inadequate. One such problem is the major acute wound, which requires cover either immediately or within 1–2 weeks after surgery (Fig. 1-2). All necrotic or potentially infected tissue must be *meticulously debrided* before the wound is covered. In more chronic situations, metal plates or prostheses can be covered (Figs. 1-14 and 1-15) and osteomyelitis treated (Figs. 1-9 through 1-13, and 1-16).

Muscle tissue is preferred in the lower extremity, and in most situations, muscle covered with split-thickness skin graft provides the best contour. Muscle tissue is also effective in filling dead space (Figs. 1-14, 1-16, and 1-17), and the infection rate is extremely low. If bulk is needed because the defect is substantial, a musculocutaneous transplant may be advantageous.

6.1.6 Amputation Stumps

If possible, the knee or elbow joint should be salvaged to provide the best ultimate function and rehabilitation. Short below-elbow or below-knee amputation stumps with wounds require good soft-tissue cover if they are to be saved. *Musculocutaneous transplants* are generally best in such situations, providing good cover over the bone stump. The cutaneous island provides additional padding and durable cover. Debulking the flap is usually needed 6 to 9 months later to decrease the mobility of the transplant once the swelling has subsided and the transplant has atrophied somewhat. A tissue expander may be used to expand the cutaneous portion of the transplant or the surrounding skin to achieve cutaneous cover over the entire stump (Fig. 1-22).

6.2 Bone

The indications for vascularized bone transplantation and the choice of transplant are considered in Chapter 3.

When bone defects occur in conjunction with major soft-tissue defects, the staging of reconstruction is important. Simultaneous soft-tissue reconstruction and bone grafting (vascularized or nonvascularized) can be performed (Fig. 3-2) early after injury or in situations where infection has not been a problem. It is safer, especially in previously infected wounds, to first provide stable soft-tissue cover, usually by muscle transplantation (Figs. 3-3 through 3-5). Thereafter, once healing without evidence of infection has been achieved, various bone grafting options can be considered.

6.3 Composite Loss (Zhong-jia 1987)

In some situations, combinations of bone, soft tissue, and toe transplants can be used to reconstruct difficult problems. The vascular pedicle of one transplant is anastomosed to the second. In this way, a fibula transplant can be combined with overlying soft tissue, or a toe can be transferred along with a cutaneous transplant. However, such procedures require a large operating team and should be reserved for the surgeon experienced in microsurgery. In addition, if vascular problems develop and the transplant does not survive, the magnitude of the loss is greater, so the patient must fully understand this risk.

6.4 Selected Bibliography

Zhong-jia Y (1987) Combined transplantation of soft tissues. Plast Reconstr Surg 79:222

Double microvascular transplants which combine bone, soft-tissue, and toe transplants are described.

7

Recipient
Site Preparation

In most circumstances, operating time can be minimized if two surgical teams work simultaneously. Two separate instrument setups are needed for transplantation to previously infected areas. Arteriograms are seldom necessary for the donor site, but they should usually be obtained for the region of the recipient site, especially if there has been previous trauma to the area. Arteriograms are not usually done in small children.

In both the leg and the forearm, it is imperative to know which vessels are supplying the foot and hand, respectively. A retrograde dorsalis pedis pulse can be diagnosed by applying pressure to occlude the posterior tibial artery while simultaneously palpating the dorsalis pedis artery. An Allen test in the hand is important. One may encounter a dominant radial artery or radial and ulnar arteries that supply separate regions (Figs. 2-1 and 1-26) (Sec. 2.9, Jones and O'Brien 1985).

The recipient vessels must be chosen and dissected with care if the need for long vein grafts is to be avoided. The most frequently used recipient vessels are listed in Table 7-1.

Table 7-1. Recipient vessels most frequently used in microvascular surgery.

Site	Recipient vessels	Site	Recipient vessels
Hand	*Radial artery* on the dorsal aspect of the hand, just before it enters between the two heads of the first dorsal interosseous muscle (end-to-side or end-to-end) (Fig. 4-19) *Common digital vessels* (Fig. 4-11) *Palmar arch* (Fig. 2-1)	Posterior knee and distal thigh (*continued*)	*Branch of the popliteal artery* to the medial gastrocnemius *Other branches of the popliteal artery* around the knee *Femoral artery* in the region of the adductor hiatus
Forearm and elbow	*Radial artery* (Figs. 3-2 and 4-4) (*Ulnar artery* occasionally)	Anterior and lateral knee, and distal thigh	In the presence of a good posterior tibial artery supplying the foot, the anterior tibial artery can be dissected into the leg, divided, and swung back and used in retrograde fashion; it may be helpful to bring the artery deep to the tibialis anterior (Fig. 1-14)
Upper arm	Branches of the *brachial artery* (microvascular soft-tissue transplants are unusual in this region)		
Heel	*Posterior tibial artery* (Fig. 1-15)		
Leg	*Anterior tibial artery* (found by following the small pedicles between the extensor hallucis longus and the extensor digitorum longus) (Figs. 1-9 and 1-12b) *Posterior tibial artery* (Fig. 1-10)	Proximal thigh	*Lateral circumflex artery* (or the pedicle to the tensor fasciae latae) *Medial circumflex artery* (or the pedicle to the gracilis)
Posterior knee and distal thigh	In the presence of a good anterior tibial artery supplying the foot, the *posterior tibial artery* can be swung back and used in retrograde fashion (Fig. 1-16)	Hip region	*Inferior epigastric artery* (Fig. 1-17) *Lateral circumflex artery* (or the pedicle to the tensor fasciae latae) *Medial circumflex artery* (or the pedicle to the gracilis)
		Spine	*Intercostal arteries* (Fig. 3-9)

If no other vessel is available, the same vessel can be used a second time for a second transplant. This strategy depends on the bed of the first transplant, which, if satisfactory, will provide adequate supply. I have used this approach on four occasions without problems, but careful judgment and caution must be exercised (Fig. 3-8). Clamping the pedicle and observing the vascularity in the transplant is wise, and other vessels should be used if available.

In few areas of surgery is failure as immediately apparent as in microvascular transplantation. Such failure represents an enormous loss to the patient. A tissue survival rate of over 95% is acceptable but cannot be achieved without a focused effort. Approximately 10–15% of transplants will need reoperation to salvage them after vascular problems arise, and these will make the difference between an acceptable and an unacceptable tissue survival rate.

Occasionally, a faulty arterial or venous repair must be redone, but this remedy is only feasible if the problem is detected very shortly after thrombosis. Far more frequently, a vein graft is required. This graft is either anastomosed to a different recipient artery or vein, or the same vessel is used more proximally, out of the zone of injury (Fig. 1-15). One of the most common causes of vascular failure results from the use of damaged vessels in this *zone of injury*. Vessels must be very carefully scrutinized under high magnification for any irregularities of the intimal lining; if these exist, the vessel must be used more proximally, even if it means having to use a vein graft.

Transplant salvage by *reoperation* is only effective if thrombosis is diagnosed *within hours* of its occurrence (Fig. 8-1). In most cases, an experienced observer can make the diagnosis of arterial or venous compromise through careful scrutiny of the transplant. However, this determination is difficult in some situations, such as if the patient is dark-skinned or very pale-skinned, or if the replanted part has been injured, macerated, or blistered. Also, an experienced observer may not always be available because of staffing or shift changes. These factors make a reliable monitor important.

The *ideal monitor* should be simple to use, continuous, quantitative, and noninvasive (Tables 8-1 and 8-2). In addition, direct monitoring of the capillary circulation in the tissue itself is preferable to monitoring the more proximal vessels. After all, it is *this* tissue that must survive for the transplant to be successful (Fig.

8-2f). Unfortunately, the ideal monitor for every transplant and every situation does not exist, but many different kinds of monitors are available. The following is my *approach* to monitoring transplants and replants.

If a skin surface is available, one of two kinds of monitors can be used. The *pulse oxymeter* (Fig. 8-2a) has all the necessary features outlined above, but it can only be used when the transmitter and receiver in the apparatus face each other. This requirement means that it can be used in toe transplants and replants of all types when it can be placed around the end of a finger (Fig. 8-2b). It cannot be used for a cutaneous transplant. The *dermal fluorimeter* (Fig. 8-2c) can be used on any skin surface, including digits or cutaneous transplants. An injection of fluorescein is administered

Table 8-1. Monitoring in microsurgery.

Type of transplant	monitor
Replant	Pulse oxymeter
Toe	Pulse oxymeter
Cutaneous	Fluorimeter
Muscle	Clinical observation; implanted temperature probe
Bone (buried)	Implanted temperature probe

Table 8-2. Comparison of the pulse oxymeter and dermal fluorimeter.

Pulse oxymeter	Dermal fluorimeter
Very simple	Simple
Reading is continuous	Read every 2 hours
Quantitative	Quantitative
Noninvasive	Requires an IV injection
Useful only on digits	Useful on all skin